Medical Tourism New Directions

Medical Tourism
New Directions

P.N. Girija Prasad

ADHYAYAN

ADHYAYAN PUBLISHERS & DISTRIBUTORS
NEW DELHI (INDIA)

Published by
ADHYAYAN PUBLISHERS & DISTRIBUTORS
4378/4B, 105, J.M.D. House, Murari Lal Street
Ansari Road, Darya Ganj, New Delhi - 110002
Ph.: 011-23263018, 011-23277156, Fax: 011-23280028
Email: adhyayanpublishers@yahoo.com

Medical Tourism New Directions

Edition 2011
ISBN 978-81-8435-292-4

Printed in India

Published by Harish Chandra Yadav for Adhyayan Publishers & Distributors, Laser Typeseting at A.V. Rao and Printed at Tarun Offset Printers, Delhi

Preface

The concept of medical tourism as a global medical market is not new phenomenon. Even in ancient times, people travelled to other countries for health related purposes. The ancient Greeks and Egyptians travelled to health resorts in the Mediterranean for purification and spiritual healing. The first recorded case of medical tourism described Greek pilgrims who travelled from the Mediterranean Sea to Epidaurus, a small territory in the Sardonic Gulf, known as sanctuary of Asclepius, the healing god. Since the 1500s India has enjoyed a rich history of providing yoga instruction as well as Ayurveda healing to patients from around the world.

There is no universally accepted definition for "medical tourism," but the phrase generally refers to travelling abroad for health care services. Medical tourism is market-driven; it is shaped by the complex interactions of myriad medical, social, economical, and political forces. Many countries are working to successfully compete in the medical tourism marketplace by advertising variety of medical, surgical and dental services in comfortable modern facilities. Cost and quality are typically the most important factors patients consider in choosing specific destinations for treatment. However, many patients also consider amenities commonly found in resorts and hotels. Medical tourists travel four corners of the world for executive health evaluations, ophthalmologic care, cosmetic dentistry, and surgery These countries have large, modern medical facilities that are staffed by well-trained physicians who perform complex procedures such as minimally invasive / off-pump heart surgery, correction of congenital cardiac abnormalities in children, thoracic organ transplantation, and implantation of mechanical cardiac devices.

Despite the long travel time involved, India is a popular destination for medical tourists. It arguably has the lowest cost and highest quality of all medical tourism destinations and English is widely spoken. The medical tourism industry offers high potential for India primarily because of its inherent advantages in terms of cost and quality. However the competition is getting heated up and the success in future will largely be determined by development and implementation of a joint strategy by various players in the industry. India is emerging as an attractive, affordable for healthcare, but there are some challenges that the country has to overcome to become a tourist destination with competent health care industry. The government should step in the role of a regulator and a facilitator of private investment in healthcare. Joint ventures with overseas partners and establishment of medicities will help in India building a significant advantage and leadership position in the industry.

This book provides well-documented and carefully organised analysis of a type of travel that is not new but which has grown and changed dramatically in the last decade. Packed with authoritative information on the current rends and new directions in this field, it is also blessedly free of jargon, making it a superb resource for both scholars and students alike.

P.N.Girija Prasad

Contents

1

Medical Tourism: Nature and Scope

The tourism industry is one of the major segments of the world economy. It is a major contributor to foreign exchange earnings provides employment to millions directly and indirectly and acts as a vehicle for infrastructure development. Recognising the importance of the tourism industry, the Government of India has taken many policy measures such as Tourism Policy 1982, Tourism Plan of Action 1992 and Tourism Policy 1997. Through these policies, the government called for effective coordination of public and private participation to achieve synergy in the development of tourism. These plans identified new forms of tourism products for taking advantage of the emerging markets. Business tourism, health tourism, rural tourism, pilgrim tourism, adventure tourism, and sustainable tourism are some of the new products devised for changing demand.

Emerging Dimensions of Tourism

Tourism will expand greatly in future mainly due to the revolution that is taking place on both the demand and supply side. The changing population structure, improvement in living standard, more disposable income, fewer working hours and long leisure time, better educated people, ageing population and more curious youth in developing the countries, all will fuel the tourism industry growth. The arrival of a large number of customers, better educated and more sophisticated, will compel the tourist industry to launch new products and brands and re-invents traditional markets. The established traditional destinations founded on sun-sea-sand products will have to re-engineer their products. They must diversify and improve the criteria for destinations and qualities of their traditional offers. Alongside beach tourism, the tourism sector will register a steady development of new products based on natural rural business, leisure and art and culture. Thus the study of new markets and emerging markets and necessity of diversified products are the basis of our strategy, which can enhance and sustain, existing and capture new markets. Let us discuss some of the new tourism products.

Health Tourism

India is promoting the hightech healing provided by its private health care sector as a tourist attraction. This budding trade in medical tourism, selling foreigners the idea of travelling to India for world-class medical treatment at lowest cost, has really got attention in the overseas market.

The Indian system of medicine, which incorporates ayurveda, yoga, sidha, unani, naturopathy and other traditional healing treatments, is very unique and exotic. This medical expertise coupled with allopathic and other modern methods become our new focus segment to project India as a Global Healing Destination. If we believe the report published by McKenzie Consultants and Confederation of Indian Industries (CII), the response is quite positive and it could be generating revenue approximately Rs.100b by the year 2012. Our medical tourism provides low cost treatment. Perhaps you will wonder that the cost of same treatment in the US is ten times more than that in India. Many state governments like Kerala, Andhra Pradesh, Uttranchal, and Karnataka have been showcasing their medical tourism segment in certain focused market like the Gulf and African regions.

Indian private sector hospitals have undertaken massive investment in the area of health. These super-speciality hospitals employ efficient and expert doctors and other paramedical staffs with modern facilities. The experienced doctors, dedicated service minded experts have made available their services for giving alternative system of medicines and treatments. Health camps, lecture training classes are also arranged for general awareness. Yogasana has become popular and widespread and many public and private and other organisations conduct Yoga classes. Ayurveda, naturopathy and nature treatments are popular around the world.

Ayurveda

India has a rich heritage in the areas of traditional and natural medicines. The earliest mention of Indian medical practices can be found in the Vedas and Samhitas of Charaka, Bhela and Shusruta. A systematic and scientific approach was adopted by the sages of the time leading to the development of a system that is relevant even today. India is the land of Ayurveda. It believes in removing the cause of illness and not just curing the disease itself. It is based on herbals and herbal components without having side effects.

Ayurveda considers that the base of life lies in the five primary elements; ether (space), air, fire, water and earth. And the individual is made up of a unique proportion of the five elements in unique combinations to form three doshas (vata, pita and kapha). When any of these doshas become acute, a person falls ill. Ayurveda recommends a special life style and nutritional guidelines supplemented with herbal medicines. If toxins are abundant, then a cleaning process known as Panchkarma is recommended to eliminate those unwanted toxins and revitalize both mind and body. Ayurveda offers treatments for ailments such as arthritis, paralysis, obesity, sinusitis, migraine, premature aging and general health care.

Kerala is a world tourist destination and part of the reasons lies with the well- known stress-releasing therapies of famed Ayurvedic research centres. The climate along with the blessing of nature has turned Kerala into the ideal place for ayurvedic, curative and rejuvenating treatments.

Yoga

If Ayurveda is the science of body, yoga is the science of the mind. Practised together they can go a long way in making an individual fit. The word yoga means to join together. The ultimate aim of yoga is to unite the human soul with the universal spirit. Yoga was developed 5000 years ago and the base of yoga is described in the Yoga Sutra of Patanjali. This describes eight stages of yoga. These are Yam (universal moral commands), Niyam (self purification), Asana (posture), Pranayama (breathing control), Prathyahara (withdrawal of mind from external objects), Dharana (concentration), Dhyana (meditation), and Samadhi (state of super-consciousness). To get the benefits of yoga, one has to practice Asana, Pranayama and Yoganidra. With the regular practice of asanas one can control cholesterol level, reduce weight, normalize blood pressure and improve cardiac performance. Pranayama helps to release tensions, develop relaxed state of mind and Yoganidra is a form of meditation that relaxes both physiological and psychological systems. Today, yoga has become popular in India and abroad and in a number of places including urban and rural areas yoga is taught and practised.

Spas

Most of the other parts of the world have their own therapies and treatment that are no doubt effective in restoring wellness and beauty. New kinds of health tours that are gaining popularity in India are spa tours. Spas offer the unique advantages of taking the best from the west and the east combining them with the indigenous system and offering best of the two worlds. In hydropathy, Swedish massages work with the Javanese Mandy, lulur, aromatherapy, reflexology and traditional ayurveda procedures to help keep the tourist healthy and enhance beauty. Combining these therapies with meditation, yoga and pranayama make the spa experience in India a new destination for medical tourism. The spas are very useful for controlling blood pressure, insomnia, cure tension, depression, paralysis and number of other deadly diseases. Ananda Resort in Rishikesh, Angsana Resort, Golden Palm Spa and Ayurgram in Bangalore offer ayurveda, naturopathy, yoga and meditation packages.

Allopathy

India has made rapid strides in advanced health care systems, which provides world-class allopathic treatment. This has become possible because of the emergence of the private sector in a big way in this field. More and more foreign tourists are realizing that India is an ideal place for stopover treatment. Indian Multi-speciality hospitals are providing world-class treatment at an amazingly economical cost as compared to the west. Quality services and low price factor primarily go in favour of

India. The cardio care, bone marrow transplantation, dialysis, kidney transplant, neuron–surgery, joint replacement surgery, urology, osteoporosis and numerous diseases are treated at Indian hospitals with full professional expertise. Apollo hospital group, Escorts in Delhi, Jason Hospital, Global Hospital, and Max Health Care are catering to medical care for international patients in the areas of diagnostic, disease management, preventive health care and incisive surgeries.

The tourism department has devised websites in order to provide information. Many Ayurveda health resorts that are owned and rum by traditional Ayurveda Institutes have come up. Ayurgram is a novel concept that not only offers heritage accommodation but also offers a whole range of Ayurvedic treatments and rejuvenating packages. Similarly hotels have also included these types of packages in their holidays. Some of the tour operators have worked out all-inclusive medical treatment package that include treatment, accommodation, food, airport transfers, post operation recuperative holidays, along with a host of other facilities.

This in fact shows our product offers true value for money for service. Many world-class state-of-the-art furnishing and equipment are being added to our Ayurveda Resorts to welcome international guests. Along with these hospitals there are many centres which offer not just physical but emotional and spiritual healing to patients. With all these India is going to be one of the leading medical health care destinations in the near future.

Spiritual Tourism

Globally people are increasingly mentally disturbed and looking for solace in spiritual reading, meditation and moments of divine ecstasy. Our country has been known as the seat of spiritualism and India's cosmopolitan nature is best reflected in its pilgrim centres. Religion is the lifeblood for followers of major religion and sects. Hinduism, Islam, Buddhism, Jainism, Zoroastrianism and Christianity have lived here for centuries. The visible outpouring of religious fervour is witnessed in the architecturally lavish temples, mosques, monasteries and Churches spreads across the length and breadth of the country. India is not only known as a place rich in its culture with varied attractions but also for many places of worship, present itself as embodiments of compassion where one get peace of mind. Thus India has been respected as a destination for spiritual tourism for domestic and international tourists. Spiritual tourism is also termed as religious heritage tourism. It includes all the religions mentioned above; religious places associated with, emotional attachment to these centres and infrastructure facilities for the tourists. This can also be referred to as pilgrimage tourism, as clients are not looking for luxury but arduous journeys to meet the divine goal or simple life.

The essence of spiritual tourism is inner feeling through love. Love should not be rationed on the basis of caste, creed and economic status or intellectual attainment of the recipient. Religions come into existence for the purpose of regulating human life; what are common to all of them are the principles of love. Thus through religious tourism there is a sincere effort to bring better understanding among various communities, nations and thus foster global unity.

Hinduism is one of the oldest religions of India. Over 5000 years of religious history created wonderful temples and survived through ages all over India. The most popular spiritual tours are those that are centred on holy Ganges River. Badrinath, Kedarnath, Haridwar, Gangotri, Yamunotri, Allahabad, Varanasi. Jaganath temple at Puri, Bhubaneshwar, Konark in Orissa, Mata Vaishnodevi of Jammu and Kashmir, are some of the important pilgrim centres in north India. There are many spiritual sites in South India as well which dates back beyond the 10th century. Rameshwaram, Mahabalipuram, Madurai Meenakshi temple in Tamilnadu and Tirupati in Andhra Pradesh are some pilgrim centres. Every year millions of tourists, both domestic and international, visit these places.

India is special to Buddhists all over the world and India is the destination for pilgrimage because Buddhism emerged in India. The country is dotted with places that are associated with the life and times of Gutham Buddha; Lumbini-the birthplace of Buddha, Saranath where Buddha delivered his first sermon, Buddha Gaya where lord Buddha attained enlightenment and Vaishali where he delivered his last sermon and announced his nirvana.

Sikhism also emerged in India. The Golden Temple in Amritsar, the Hemkund Sahib, and Gurunanak Devji Gurudwara at Manikaran, which is also known for its hot water springs with healing properties, the holy city of Patna Sahib and Anandpur Sahib are important for Sikhs.

The Jain temples of Dilwara and Mount Abu in Rajasthan, the Gomateswara temple at Karnataka, draw thousands of Jain followers. Even small communities like the Bahais have their own Lotus Temple at Delhi.

The Sultanate and Moghul empires built many historical monuments and mosques during their reign, all over the country. Red Fort, Fatehapur Sikri, Jama Masjid, TajMahal, Charminar etc., bear testimony to the blend of the Indian and Islam traditions of architecture. The followers of Islam have many mosques and shrines of Sufi Saints, like Moin-Uddin Chisti and Nizamuddin Aulia. For Christians, spiritual tours to Goa among other place like Mumbai and Kolkata are must. Among the most popular sites in Goa is the church of Our Lady of Rosary, the Rachel Seminary, and Church of Bom Jesus.

In addition to pilgrim centres there are personalities like the Satya Sai Baba, Osho, Shirdhi and others. This shows that spirituality and religion in India is a serious pursuit. The State Governments concerned, charitable trusts, temple trusts have made elaborate arrangements for accommodation, transport and ritual ceremonies. These organizations are also running hospitals, educational institutes, ashrams, meditation centres which benefit local community. More than 500 religious places have been identified and efforts are being made to develop these centres by Central and State Governments with private participation.

Mice Tourism

The meetings, incentives, conferences and exhibitions (MICE) industry is extensively and rapidly growing and is largely associated with travel for business purpose. MICE related events include meetings, conferences, conventions, exhibitions and incentive travels. Each of these different subsections of MICE has quite different characteristics although the industry is often referred to as MICE. Increasingly convention bureaus serve the needs of meetings, incentives and exhibitions organizers and service providers supply each of the sectors.

Business Tourism

With the Indian economy opening up and government restrictions loosening, Mumbai, Bangalore, Hyderabad, Chennai, Delhi and Kolkata are assuming importance as major centres of business activity in the country. The days of red- tape always associated with Indian business activity is a thing of the past and corporate India has moved towards more western standards of professionalism. Since the liberalization of the Indian economy, MICE tourism is becoming a growing segment in India. More and more business people have been coming to India for business purpose and adding business with pleasure in their India tour.

Most of the hotels and tour operators offer special facilities for travellers; some even specialized in this field. They offers pick-up at the airport, corporate floor rooms which will feature phones, fax machines, computers, journals. All rooms offer elaborate conferencing facilities at hotels and special conventions centres. Hotels are adept in organizing theme banquets for a product launch, small cocktails etc. The important conference centres are New Delhi, Mumbai, Jaipur, Kovalam, Chennai, Bangalore, Agra, and Goa where popular convention tours offer exciting possibilities.

Incentive Tourism

Incentive travel has emerged as a popular means of rewarding the employees' achievements and contributions, by several business houses especially multinational companies, Insurance Companies, Banks, Pharmaceuticals Firms, etc. Employees are given free tickets or holidays packages to select destinations all paid by company. These are given as added perks to keep up the interest of the executives who are the high performers of the company. Incentive tours market has become fast growing sector within the tourism industry.

Adventure Tourism

Youth tourism has been identified as one of the largest segments of global and domestic tourism. The young travellers are primarily experience seekers, collecting, enquiring unique experiences. Adventure and risk have a special role to play in the behaviour and attitudes of young travellers. The growing number of young travellers is being fuelled by a number of factors such as increased participation in higher education, falling level of youth unemployment, increased travel budget through parental contribution, search for an even more exciting and unique experience and cheaper long distance travel. Youth and adventure tourism appears to have considerable growth potential. The rising income in some major potential source markets such as the Central and Eastern Europe, Asia and Latin America, combined with the lower travel cost, growing student populations around the world particularly in developing countries, has fuelled the demand.

India has been an attraction for travellers from all over the world. Though in the field of international tourism, the segment of adventure tourism in India is getting only a fraction of such traffic. The trend has been showing an increased movement year after year with the development of facilities and greater awareness about adventure tourism options. Indian tourism offers both international and domestic adventurers a wide choice of adventures. Water sports, elephant safari, skiing, yachting, hail-skiing, gliding, sailing, tribal tours, orchid tours, scaling the high peaks of Himalayas, trekking to the valley of flowers, riding the waves in rapids, and camel safari in the deserts are breath taking opportunities for nature enthusias. Ladakh, the Garwal hills, the Himachal hills, Darjeeling, Goa, Lakshadweep, Andaman and Nicobar, Jaisalmer and wildlife sanctuaries and reserves are some of the places that offer adventure tourism.

Himalayas are the centre of India's main adventure activities as well as outdoor recreational tourism. Our rivers, backwaters, Indian Ocean, Arabian Sea and deserts are unique attractions for the various branches of adventure. Trekking holds out the greatest potential in terms of numbers. It requires little infrastructure and carries its benefits to remote hills and mountain regions. Many of them are economically poor and backward. For our own youth it also helps in inculcating a spirit of adventure, respect for nature. Indian Mountaineering Federation, Ministry of Tourism and State Governments are trying to improve trekking facilities and ensure safety and protection of travellers. The Institute of Mountaineering also organises courses for guides to train them in basic rock climbing safety procedures, environmental knowledge, and flora and fauna conservation. The major trek heads in the Himalayan region include Kashmir valley, Kirshwasser Zanskar, Ladhak, Lahul and Spiti, Champa and Manali, etc, Trekking in the Himalayas is a quite enjoyable. Let us now discuss some important adventure activities:

Mountaineering Expedition

This is the first and foremost activity in the Himalayas. In India, the expeditions are controlled and regulated by Indian Mountaineering Federation, which is the nodal body. Foreign expedition groups have to request the Indian Mountaineering Foundation (IMF) to book the required peak and IMF confirms the peak, by charging the royalty depending upon the number of persons and height of peak. Ministry of Defence, Home Ministry, Ministry of External Affairs are also involved in this process.

River Rafting

The Himalayan river's offer River rafting that run through the beautiful terrains, sandy white beaches, boulder studded rapids, river confluences, deep gorges, and some revered temples and towns. White-water sports are popular in Rishikesh, Manali, Zanskar Teesta, Beas, Central Ministry of Tourism has great extremely extended support to import inflatable rafts, canoes, kayaks, and accessories to boost water sports. Lakshadweep and Andaman have been promoted for scuba diving and windsurfing.

Water Sports

To boost water sports, water skiing and sailing both in seas and lakes, and river facilities has been provided. Chilka Lake in Orissa, Kollam in Kerala, Bhopal Lake in Madhya Pradesh, Dal Lake in Kashmir are some of the places where facilities have been provided for water sports. In Himachal hills Heli-skiing is also being promoted in season. The Garwal Mandal Vikas Nigam provides regular skiing courses during the season. It can be said that India is a new destination for adventure tourism. The Ministry of tourism, The Himalayan Task Force and Himalayan Tourism and Adventure Tourism Board (HMTAB) meet every year to discuss conservation, promotion for Himalayan tourism, and conservation of ecology.

Nature Tourism

In search of new tourism products, travellers and suppliers are today seeking to reshape the meaning of nature as a tourism attraction. Modern nature based tourism focuses on experiencing flora and fauna in natural settings. The nature based tourism related to nature, its attractiveness so that the visitors experience it in its natural settings. Eco-tourism takes into account unspoiled natural and sociocultural attraction. Today the term nature tourism is often used synonymously with eco-tourism. Today nature tourism is the fastest growing segment of the tourism sector. It comprises around 40-60% of all international tourism.

Diversity of India is to be seen not only in its people, culture, religions, language and life style, the diversity starts in the land itself. The snowbourd peaks of the Himalayas, tropical rain forests, and hot deserts and breathtaking beautiful coasts. Each diverse geographical region generates a different picture and exploring them provides a unique experience. Now all these are packaged for tourists to provide eco-friendly holidays in India.

Wild Life

The diversity of wild life in India is as rich as that of its flora and fauna. The great wealth of Indian wildlife can be imagined with the sight of majestic elephants, the dance of peacocks, the camel strides, the roar of tigers, at unparalleled acts of beauty. Watching birds and animals in their natural habitat is an experience in itself. The vastness of wild life and wilderness is India unparallel in the world. All these account for the immense opportunities for wild life tourism in India. The immense heritage of wild life in India comprises 80 national parks and another whopping 441 wild life sanctuaries including bird sanctuaries. These reserves and forest areas are spread across the breadth and length right form the foot hills of Himalayan, the Jim Corbet National park to six national parks in Andaman, from Ranthambhor national park in Rajasthan to Hazaribag wild life sanctuary in Bihar. India also boasts of the unique ecosystem at Sunderbans which is a UNESCO world heritage site and home to the largest number of tigers in the world.

The Himalayan region is renowned for being the national habitat for a variety of wild life, elephants, snow leopards, deer, panther, wild buffalos, wild ass, one horned rhinoceros, porcupine, snow leopards, etc. The Kaziranga Game Sanctuary is ideal habitat for the rhino that the nature lovers and environmentalists are fascinated by. The great Indian bustard and the black buck of Kerera sanctuary attract a lot of tourists. The Madhav National Park (Shivpuri Park) is another rich habitat for the wild life. The royal animal, tiger happens to be symbol of strength and speed. Amongst the best-known tiger reserves in India is Bandhawgarh in Madhya Pradesh. It is also known as the crown in the wild life heritage of India.

The variety of birds in India is enormous. Several hundred species of bird can be spotted across India. Indian wild life has its share of native birds along with migratory birds. The region of Andaman is home to rare species of birds like Narcondum hornbills, Nicobar pigeons and megaspores. The Himalayan region is well known as the natural habitat for the pheasant griffon, vulture and ravens. Dudhuwa wild life reserve, Keoladeao, Ghana national park, the Bharatpur bird sanctuary in Rajasthan is home to indigenous and migratory water birds. These bird sanctuaries are attracting tourists from far and wide.

Fishing and Angling

Among the amazing array of nature tours offered in India are those that offer angling and fishing. The waters of Indian subcontinent are mind-blowing grounds for the nature sports. The adventures settings range form the majestic Himalayan valleys, snow fed streams and high altitude lakes and wide coastal stretches of the Arabia Seas and Bay of Bengal. Amidst the beautiful hills of the Himalayas is tented accommodation along the river beds, excellent option for adventure holidays in India. The Cauvery fishing lodge near Mysore, the hill stations of Munnar, and streams and lakes of Kerala and Kashmir are a paradise for anglers.

Hill Stations

At heights that range from 600 m to 3500m above sea level, most of the hill resorts of India are tourist destination in India. The hill stations add to the nature tour of India with majestic mountains and ravishing rivers. Mountain ranges of Shimla, Kullu Manali, Dalhousie, Palampur in Himachal Pradesh, Nainital-Almora-Kausani in Kumaon hills of Uttar

Pradesh, Pachmarhi in MadhyaPradesh, Darjeeling are important for their snow-dusted peaks, lakes, parks and hot springs. The waterfalls, sulphur bath and all provide such an experience, which will linger in one's mind.

Green heavens are on not only in the forest but the Islands are also a source of the best eco-tourism destinations. The tourism activities in Lakshadweep bring you close to nature. Andamans that are covered with rainforest, ringed by coral reefs, marine life, swimming and sunbathing are good experiences.

We are promoting tourism but while promoting tourism in eco-sensitive areas the emphasis is to control the volume of tourists so that the fragile balance of the area is not disturbed. The whole objective of nature tourism is to have purposeful travel to natural areas. Taking special note of this very objective of the eco-tourism while utilising the economic opportunities we should ensure conservation of natural resources. People travel to those areas, which enlightens, educates and entertains them. The new changed concept of nature tourism revives the tired source of the eco-tourism. It also provides basic economic upliftment to local people and other stakeholders who are directly dependent on this natural heritage. This strong relationship is targeted throughout eco-tourism.

Rural Tourism

Rural tourism has been identified as one of the priority areas for development of Indian tourism. Rural tourism experience should be attractive to the tourists and sustainable for the host community. The Ninth Plan identified basic objectives of rural tourism as:

— Improve the quality of life of rural people

— Provide good experience to the tourist

— Maintain the quality of environment.

Indian villages have the potential for tourism development. With attractive and unique traditional way of life, rich culture, nature, crafts, folklore and livelihood of Indian villages are a promising destination for the tourist. It also provides tourism facilities in terms of accessibility, accommodation, sanitation and security. Rural tourism can be used as a means to:

— Improve the well being of the rural poor
— Empower the rural people
— Empower the women
— Enhance the rural infrastructure
— Participate in decision-making and implementing tourism policies
— Interaction with the outside world
— Improve the social condition of lower sections of the society.
— Protection of culture, heritage, and nature.

To tap the immense opportunities, coordinated actives of all agencies involved in the development are required. A carefully planned and properly implemented development will definitely benefit the community economically and improve the quality of life in the villages. The success of such development depends upon the people's participation at grass root level for the development of tourist facilities and for creating a tourist friendly atmosphere. Development of rural tourism is fast and trade in hotels and restaurants is growing rapidly. Increase in the share of earnings through rural tourism will no doubt; provide an attractive means of livelihood to the poor rural community. It increases the purchasing power at all levels of community and strengthens the rural economy. Development of infrastructure facilities such as rail, electricity, water, health and sanitation will definitely improve the quality of life.

Sustainable Tourism

The concept of sustainability means that mankind must live within the capacity of the environment that supports. Sustainable development has been defined briefly as "that which meets the needs of the present without compromising the ability of future generations to meet their own needs". The definition brings out certain important aspects of sustainable tourism:

— Conservation and enhancement of resources for the future generation
— Protection of biological diversity
— Equity within and between generations

— Integration of environmental, social and economic considerations

The concept of sustainable development is all about conservation and stewardship of resources for the future. The support for ecologically sustainable development emerging strongly in the tourism sector, as it is the logical way of balancing environmental concerns with growth and development of the industry. Environmental problems facing the world today are of such magnitude that urgent actions have to be taken at the highest levels to counter this fatal degradation. But it is not just enough for government organisations to work towards sustainable development. Every individual, every neighbourhood, and every community has to contribute in every away possible to get close to the goal. Since the earth summit, the concept of sustainable development has been placed firmly on the global agenda. This issue is assuming great significance in the development of tourism in India also.

Tourism activities depend upon nature and natural heritage, it is essential to ensure that tourism development is ecologically sustainable ecological process must not be neglected. Similarly tourism offers real experience of unique culture of the country. Hence the development should ensure that social and cultural sustainable tourism development compatible with the culture and values of the local people.

The World Tourism Organization (WTO) defined sustainable tourism development as "that which meets the needs of present tourist and host regions while protecting and enhancing opportunities for the future. It is envisaged as leading to the management of all resources in such a way that economic, social and aesthetic needs can be fulfilled while maintaining cultural integrity, essential for ecological process, biological diversity and life supporting system".

Thus tourism has to be human and adapted to the needs of the tourist, respond to the needs of the local communities, be socioeconomic and culturally well planned and environmentally sound. The tourism must offer products that are operated in harmony with the local environment, community attitudes and culture so that they become permanent beneficiaries and not the victims of tourism. The basic cultural identity of these local people should not be adversely affected. Sustainability also ensures economically sustainable-development process in the efficient management of resources and such management to ensure that the resource supports the future as well as the present generation.

Thus sustainable tourism aims to:

- Improve the quality of life of people.
- Provide good experience to the tourists
- Maintain the quality of environment that is essential for both tourists and the local community.

Tourism can be one of the effective tools for building a prosperous community economically, socially and culturally. It must be environmentally sustainable and based on the sustainance of the natural and cultural base. Each destination should examine whether it has adequate attractions and facilities for tourism and there is a potential for tourism generating markets to be open to exploitation. The carrying capacity is the central principle in environmental protection and sustainable tourism development. It determines the maximum use of any place without causing negative effects on resources on community, economy and culture. Thus tourism has to be environmentally sustainable in both natural and cultural environment

Nature of Medical and Healthcare Tourism

Travel itself exposes travellers to various mental and physical challenges in their new environment as part of their experience. This is especially so when the medical tourist is ill and debilitated and, therefore, more susceptible to contracting illnesses from the destinations. However, the cost benefit for the travelling medical tourist to receive medical treatment often compensates for this travel risk at the destination.

There are numerous definitions of tourists. However, it is accepted that tourists are travellers who have travelled and stayed away from their home environment for 24 hours or more, and hence, have often utilised some form of accommodation facility. Those travellers who do not meet this 24 hour criterion are generally referred to as 'visitors'. For travellers that travel overseas for medical purposes, conceptually, they would meet the definition of a tourist. Since medical tourists are travellers whose main motivation for travel is for a specific purpose, medical tourists can be categorised as a group of special interest tourists, hence participating in a form of special interest tourism. There is no one definition for medical tourism but it is generally accepted that this term is used to refer to travel activity that involves a medical procedure or activities that promote the wellbeing of the tourist. Figure 1 illustrates the components of medical and healthcare tourism.

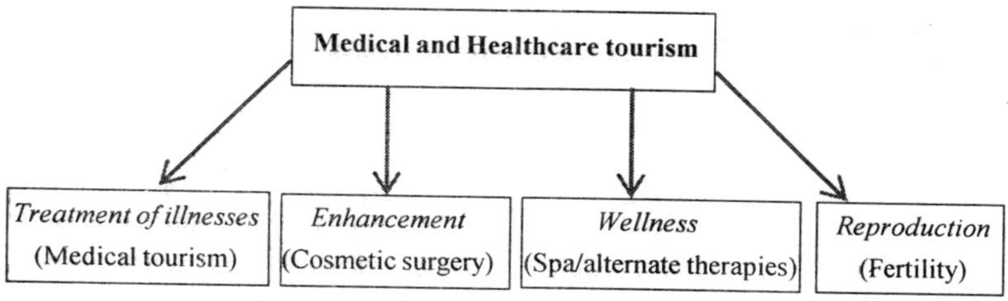

Figure 1. Medical and healthcare tourism and components

The term 'treatment of illnesses', generally includes medical checkups, health screening, dental treatment, joint replacements, heart surgery, cancer treatment, neurosurgery, transplants and other procedures that require qualified medical intervention. These can range from healthcare services that can be provided by a local general practitioner to complex surgical procedures such as transplants.

'Enhancement' procedures are carried out mainly for aesthetic purposes. Some of these procedures require qualified medical personnel but much of this work is non-disease related (unless disfigurement is caused by disease). Examples of such procedures include all cosmetic surgery, breast surgery, face-lifts, liposuction and cosmetic dental work.

This component of the tourism and healthcare tourism is traditionally most associated with the tourism and leisure industry. The 'wellness' segment of medical and healthcare tourism promotes healthier lifestyles. Therefore, these products can include treatment in spas, thermal and water treatments, acupuncture, aromatherapy, beauty care, facials, exercise and diet, herbal healing, homeopathy, massage, spa treatment, yoga and other similar products. There is normally no need for a qualified doctor to provide these services, although many professionals providing these services, are often accredited members of the various associations.

'Reproduction' tourism is an increasing and growing area of medical tourism travel. Under this component, there are patients who seek fertility-related treatments such as in vitro and in vivo fertilization and other similar procedures. In some situations, the travel is motivated and influenced by the legislation in the country of origin and host country. Some fertility procedures are illegal in some countries. Furthermore, 'birth tourism' is also included in this category. This category involves a pregnant mother who travels to another country to give birth to her baby in order to utilise the services, which are often free. In addition, a further advantage for her is to have her child gain citizenship of the new country and thus be able to reside permanently in the new location. At times, potential parents travel for the purposes of adopting children because the legislation and supply of babies for adoption is easier in host countries.

International Medical Tourism and Porter's Diamond

Porter's diamond of national competitive advantage is a modern international trade theory. It was derived and used to conceptualise the four conditions that are important when conducting international business. These four factors originate from earlier country and firm-based theories. In simple terms, the country based theories relate to the international trade theories of nations as a unit of business and the firm-based theories are those which relate to the firm as a unit of business. International business can be defined as commerce or business involving one of more countries and/or businesses located in a different country. In either situation, it involves cross border or trans-border commercial activities, hence including the complexities arising in different legislation, political environments, cultures, societies and other factors. As medical tourism generally involves the participation and activities of people and transactions in more than one country, this is appropriately relevant to international business.

Originally, Porter's diamond of national competitive advantage was developed from the observations of the practices of about one hundred international businesses across ten different countries. Therefore, many of the components would encompass and consider most of the elements that are essential for the strategic decision-making of a firm intending to conduct international business. In the shape of a two dimensional diamond, four main components are included in this model (Figure 2). These include factor conditions, demand conditions, related and supporting industries, and firm strategy, structure and rivalry. Two additional, elements, which refer to chance and government, were later included in the conceptualisation to recognise the importance of these two additional components in the influence of international business.

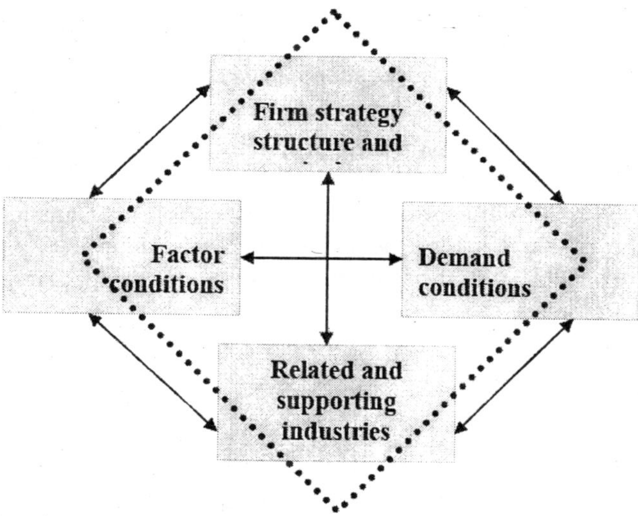

Figure 2. Porter's diamond of national competitive advantage

Factor Conditions

With factor conditions, many medical tourism products are located in warm, pleasant environments. Therefore, the basic factors, which include ideal climatic conditions, natural resources and geographic location, are an advantage for medical tourism especially for those visitors from colder climates. In addition to these basic factors, there are advanced factors that have assisted in the development of medical tourism. These include investments made by people, who usually offer medical tourism services, predominantly in private hospitals (companies) and governments. Other advanced factors include the utilisation of the worldwide web resources for the communication and marketing of the medical tourism product internationally. In terms of quality, it is said that there is little difference in the medical tourism services offered in the advanced western countries and those in the eastern or developing countries. Quite often, medial doctors and their staff are trained in western countries, have worked in western hospitals and then returned to their country of origin (eastern or developing countries) for various personal reasons. Furthermore, the recruitment of foreign-trained doctors by these private hospitals, plus attractive work conditions have helped to staff these hospitals with well-qualified people. Therefore, the quality of such healthcare services are equivalent and the services far better than that found in the hospitals in developed countries.

Labour, in a large population, is relatively cheap in developing industries. Therefore, many of the activities involved in financing a hospital can be managed at a cheaper cost because salaries are generally lower and, in turn, the savings are passed along to the patient who pays much less for the same healthcare service than that found in their home country.

Demand Conditions

As the ageing population increases, there is increasing demand for medical services, and, quite often, this demand cannot be met in many western countries under the public healthcare service. For much of the population, private healthcare is too expensive and so patients are placed onto public waiting lists for medical treatment. As these lists get longer and the price of healthcare increases, it is logical that alternative measures, which can serve this necessary demand, will be supported to improve the quality of life of these patients. Quite often, simply the cost of an expensive holiday could finance medical treatment and a recuperative break away in the destination country. This is very attractive for many people. Both physical and mental well-being are addressed. The former is taken care of by surgical procedures, the latter involves recuperation and pampering in an exotic location that can promote mental health and wellbeing during this process. Hence, such a medical tourism experience is very attractive.

A further demand for medical tourism is created by the increasing population that do not subscribe to private healthcare insurance. There are various reasons why some people do not have medical insurance these are usually cost-related. Consequently, this would be a group of patients who would either benefit from medical tourism, or, not be able to afford any treatment at all.

Insurance companies that have to pay for the cost of medical treatment of their insured clients are continuously seeking ways of reducing their expenses and improving their services. These companies are gradually creating a demand for medical tourism as well. Where companies allow flexible claims for healthcare services, these companies may pay a smaller amount of compensation to their clients who have paid less for their medical treatment received overseas. For example, India has targeted the National Health Service to explore the use of medical services overseas. Such international business arrangements are somewhat like a sophisticated form of subcontracting or off-shoring of services, which is a commonly utilised business strategy to reduce costs.

Supporting Industries

Since medical tourism involves a form of travel to a foreign location, there is demand for some form of accommodation in the hospital or in a hotel and also for local travel at the destination. Therefore, medical tourism relies upon a developed infrastructure. The tourism industry includes the provision of travel by the airlines and accommodation in hotels and motels and also taxis for local travel. Furthermore, there are activities that cater for the leisure and recreation of tourists, which can provide ideal facilities for a relaxing and pampered recovery from any medical procedures. With such sound infrastructures in place in most developing countries, not much further infrastructure investment is required by local businesses and host governments. In addition, foreign governments are aware that the value of the tourism dollar can be increased by the introduction and support of medical tourism and so have supported businesses investing in this new industry. Furthermore, it is recognised that a medical tourist rarely travels alone.

It is common for another relative to accompany the patient and, therefore, the accompanying person or entire family may travel to the selected destination and stay for the necessary duration of the medical treatment. Governments further encourage medical tourism by allowing visas to be easily obtained and so do not hinder the process.

Company Strategy

This factor shifts from the macro-related (at country level) toward those at micro level (at level of the firm) in the Porter's diamond. At micro level, the future of individual enterprises (including hospitals) participating in medical tourism will be dependent on their strategy, structure and rivalry. Although medical tourism is supported by governments, as with other tourism businesses, those companies, which do not provide a quality service and maintain a good customer satisfaction rating, cannot remain sustainable in the market environment. As medical tourism becomes more attractive to many countries, there will be much more international competition and rivalry. Therefore, with medical treatment being equal across many countries, the tourist would begin to select their target destination based on other reasons. Some medical enterprises have compiled packages to make it easier for tourists who then do not need to spend so much time in researching their travel and accommodation requirements. With the medical tourism facilities increasing in demand over time, as with other international business operations, there is room for multinational enterprises that can offer such healthcare services internationally. With a multinational enterprise comprising staff that is recruited internationally, there are facilities within the structure of the firm to enable these enterprises to expatriate medical staff to manage future subsidiaries around the world. Although doctors are required by law to register with the local medical associations before they can practice in the local environment, there is no such requirement for the CEO to manage and start such operations in any country. Thus, it will not be unusual in the near future to have different forms of entry modes in medical tourism, such as with franchising agreements or joint ventures.

Table 1 lists a range of countries that are currently offering international medical tourism healthcare services. This table shows that almost all the countries in the world offer some form of medical tourism services. As the benefits of medical tourism is realised in financial terms and for the wellbeing of the patients, more resources from governments and private investors in this industry will be provided.

Table 1. International medical tourism provision of service

Argentina	Czech Republic	Mexico
Australia	Dubai	Netherlands
Bahrain	France	Oman Peru
Bangladesh	Germany	Philippines
Barbados	Greece	Poland
Belgium	Hungary	Romania
Brazil	India	Russia
Bulgaria	Iran	Saudi Arabia
Canada	Israel	South Africa
Cayman Islands	Japan Jordan	Switzerland
Chile	Korea	Taiwan
Costa Rica	Lebanon	Thailand
Cuba	Lithuania	Turkey
Cyprus	Malaysia	

Scope of Medical Tourism

As with all rapid developments, there will be some need to regulate and monitor institutions in order to ensure and maintain the health and safety of medical tourists. It is more likely that this process will be reactive to issues and problems rather than pro-active in preventing problems from emerging. With some medical tourism procedures, such as heart surgery, hip replacements, cochlear implants and dental surgery, it is necessary to be aware of the qualifications and training of surgeons, operating teams and the reputation of the medical facilities offering the treatments. It cannot be taken for granted that the same level of health standards apply in the domestic and international environment. Nevertheless, the utilisation of overseas health services is not too different from the better known subcontracting or the off-shoring of services, such as those used in call centres and other business services. Since medical tourism decisions are sometimes based on higher costs and average expertise in the domestic situation, medical tourism is likely to be the new global trend for providing medical services through necessity rather than choice for many future medical tourists.

With the range and scope of medical procedures offered in the international marketplace, different countries offer different levels of control over their domestic medical tourism services. This can be risky and dangerous. In the worst case scenario, either post operative recovery does not go well and patients need to prolong their stay at the destination and therefore incur additional costs, or, if patients have returned home, they would have to seek further medical care and treatment in their home country. This would increase the cost of the overall treatment for their condition especially for cosmetic procedures, which are monitored less. Hence, 'buyers beware' is currently the norm than the exception. Therefore, in the early days of global investment in this new product, the monitoring or accreditation of these products can significantly increase their international demand. The way forward is towards some form of international monitoring of the global medical tourism product and services at governmental and global levels. This would require a large degree of international coordination and cooperation between the nations beyond that exhibited by the current day situation.

References

Bennett, M.; King, B. and Milner, L. (2004). "The health resort sector in Australia: A positioning study", *Journal of Vacation Marketing.* vol.10, no.2, pp.122-137.

CBS (2004). "Medical tourism: Need surgery, will travel", *CBS News Indepth*: healthcare, June 18,2004.

Douglas, N., Douglas, N. and Derrett, R. (2001). *Special Interest Tourism*, Wiley, Australia

Fisher, G.; Hughes, R.; Griffin, R. and Pustay, M. (2006). *International Business* Prentice Hall, Frenchs Forest.

Garcia-Altes, M. (2005). "The development of health tourism services", *Annals of Tourism Research*, vol.32, no.1,pp.222-266.

Henderson, J.C. (2004). "Healthcare tourism in Southeast Asia", *Tourism Review International*, vol.7, pp.111-121.

2

Extent and Directions of Medical Tourism

The ultimate concept of medical tourism is a tour to surrounding destination, medical treatment and savings. People from advanced countries, including the United States and Europe, see a benefit in travelling to developing third world countries, like India, Thailand, Philippines, South Africa, etc.while combining medical treatments with inexpensive vacation. The medical tourism industry offers high potential for countries like India primarily because of its inherent advantages in terms of cost and quality. However the competition is getting heated up and the success in future will largely be determined by development and implementation of a joint strategy by various players in the industry.

The increased use of medical care in one state by the residents of another state has been the result of a number of developments related to increasing globalization and interdependence. Some of the factors include the approximately 200 million persons and their families who now live in countries other than their country of birth, the increase in tourism in general, the internationalization of accredited Western style medical facilities which both attract visitors and retain nationals, the low cost of obtaining information and marketing alternative care, the existence of gaps or delays in coverage in sending countries and significant cost advantages in receiving countries. The aging of populations in Europe, North America and Asia has led to an increased demand for many procedures to treat chronic disease conditions. At the same time, in the face of increased evidence of cost savings, many who might benefit from services abroad do not do so because of the lack of coverage for such care either through public or private insurance.

There are a number of estimates and rough guesses about the number of persons utilizing and money spent on cross border medical care. A crude, but probably inflated, estimate might be one percent of total medical expenses of more than $5 trillion globally which would amount to more than $50 billion a year. But there is a wide variation in what is considered to qualify for inclusion in this figure. The wide divergence in recent estimates by Deloitte and by McKinsey Consulting of demand by US residents for medical services abroad illustrates this point. Deloitte Center for Health Solutions stated that in "2007, an estimated 750,000 Americans traveled abroad for medical care ....and this number is estimated to increase to six million by 2010." The projections used by Deloitte seem to be based on an assumption of almost geometric growth. McKinsey studied more than 20 medical travel destinations and conducted interviews with providers, patients, and intermediaries in 20 countries and concluded that 60,000 to 85,000 inpatients a year constituted the market internationally for all source countries. This excluded patients who had emergencies when travelling for other reasons, patients who travelled for outpatient care, patients who travelled for wellness such as acupuncture and massage and also international patients receiving care in their country of residence and patients who sought care in a nearby country. McKinsey contends that the current number of US residents going abroad for inpatient care only amounts to about 5-10,000 but that with insurance coverage these services the numbers of travelers from the US could increase to as much as 500-750,000 annually.

Growth in Facilities and Services

There has been rapid development of modern, well funded hospitals in a number of countries—in many cases with the participation of leading US referral hospitals and medical schools. Many of these hospitals have also sought and obtained Joint Commission International certification as a measure of quality to reassure those who now will stay in the country for care as well as to attract medical tourists.Most of these hospitals were developed to serve domestic demand for high quality medical services and to reduce the cost of paying for care abroad. In India where there is a significant and growing middle class and where there is concern for chronic disease problems there is a strong demand for these facilities. A recent study comparing Indian cardiac hospitals such as Escorts to heart surgery in the US argued that the quality seemed to be comparable although the relative cost was $6,000 in India compared to $100,000 in the US. It argued that in India the pricing has to be low enough to be affordable to the large Indian market and so a number of efficiencies have been adopted. With India in particular there has long been a large Indian population working in the Gulf, in East Africa, Britain, and the US which often returns to India for medical care.

In the Emirates where all citizens are guaranteed access to high quality care it is expected that far fewer trips abroad for care will be approved now that there are a number of first class hospitals located there. Similarly in Saudi Arabia there has been a concerted effort to develop high quality tertiary facilities in many parts of the kingdom. Most of the investment in these facilities is domestic—the US partners are generally medical schools or hospitals and do not provide capital. The Christus hospital system in the US has entered into a partnership with a group in Mexico and owns and manages a chain of hospitals in Mexico. Since the enterprise is nonprofit they finance low income clinics and services in Mexico with the proceeds of the partnership. Apollo hospitals in India and the Parkway hospital system in Singapore have also developed hospitals in a number of other countries including Bangladesh.

Traditional Chinese medicine and Ayuravedic medicine and acupuncture are all therapies that are increasingly popular in the west. China, India, Thailand, and Malaysia attract tourists, people who wish to be trained in these therapies and disciplines and patients who are seeking a cure or at least improved functioning. Two major Chinese hospitals offering traditional Chinese Medicine include Beijing TCM hospital of China and Guilin TCM hospital of China. Similarly there are Ayuravedic spas and treatment centers throughout much of India. In particular there are a number in Kerala and the state of Kerala has been working to regulate and rate Ayurvedic resorts. China and India are no longer the exclusive source of such therapies. In fact there are many practitioners in the United States for example and there are a number of certified schools and training programs in traditional Chinese Medicine, acupuncture, and Ayuraveda. A US nurse rehabilitated from a stroke in a northern Chinese hospital for five months where she received an intensive regimen of deep massage, acupuncture, herbal medication, steam therapy and exercise. The total cost was about $20,000—far less than it would have been in the US. She was so pleased with the results that she has started a company connecting people with practitioners in China In the last two years or so the international availability of lower cost but good quality medical and hospital services, their quality, and relative cost have become better publicized in the United States by Time, US News and major daily newspapers.

For example, a four page set of articles in the Los Angeles Times on November 1 2008 examined not only the various options abroad but also many intermediary firms and services available to persons interested in travelling abroad for medical services. The intermediary firms range from individual websites based in an exporting country that support and promote one or two facilities to firms that provide a wider choice of facilities, arrange travel, arrange lodging at the exporting country, or help coordinate after care and other services. Other firms may provide research and others may just offer Travelocity or hotels.com style web resources to potential clients. Some are paid by the facilities, some receive fees from clients served, and some receive payment based on hits. Also, at least two trade associations have developed to represent providers and intermediaries and to promote medical tourism.

Persons Consuming Care Abroad

An earlier study delineated a number of categories of consumers who go abroad for health services as well as some other categories of consumers who may be abroad for other purposes but who consume health services when abroad. These categories included:

1. Consumers who travel abroad for medical care (whose motives include seeking higher quality, lower cost, or faster treatment, or to return to their native society, or to receive services unavailable or illegal in their nation of residence);
2. Tourists who incidentally need care abroad;
3. Retirees abroad (who often have coverage in another country and who may have retired abroad for the cost or amenities, and who

may be either native to the country to which they retire or the country from which they have coverage);

4. Temporary or migrant workers;
5. Cross border commuters who may have multinational coverage options; and
6. Residents of multinational areas with integrated health systems.

It would be a mistake to dismiss all of the categories save the first since each contributes to services being delivered to either foreign residents or residents with foreign coverage. And in the case of retirees abroad if they are forced to return home to receive covered care their consumption is not usually recorded as being delivered to a foreign resident although it is.

Consumers Who Travel Abroad

Consumers who travel abroad include those who cannot afford the care in their country of residence, those who cannot obtain that care by staying at home, and those who seek higher quality care than is available. Others may seek to travel abroad for anonymity or cultural or linguistic comfort. For those who are uninsured and for those who have an extended wait for care they deem essential and for many who are uninsured for a particular procedure cost becomes a real consideration. Table 1 which is taken from the HealthBase website seems to be fairly representative of the estimates of relative costs of specific procedures for which one is likely to travel overseas.

Traditionally services such as dental care or plastic surgery have been candidates for travelers for care because these are often not covered by health insurance. Typically however the traveler travels to a fairly nearby location as with US residents of border states who go to Mexico or many Europeans who go to Hungry for dental care or plastic surgery. It is relatively recently that people, other than those who live on or near a border with a lower income country, went abroad for relatively major surgeries and procedures in order to save money. Most of the procedures listed in Table 1 offer a sufficient spread in cost for a prospective patient to be able to afford airfare for themselves and possibly another as well as to cover the cost of a hotel room during recuperation.

Table 1. Medical Tourism-Overseas Surgery

Procedure (US$)	USA	Singapore	Thailand	India
Total Hip Replacemant	24,000	15.000	10.000	6,300
Hip Resurfacing	48,000	14,000	10,000	7.000
Breast Augmentation	10,000	8,000	3.150	2,200
Breast Reduction	10,000	8,000	3,919	3,000
Eyelid Surgery	7.000	3,750	1,413	2,200
Face Lift	20,000	6,250	4,799	3,100
Nose Surgery	7,300	4.375	3,839	1,800
Tummy Tuck	8,500	6,250	4,052	3,400
Coronary Angiography	6.000	1,313	1,250	560
Coronary Angioplasty	41,000	11,250	4,150	3,500
Coronary-artery Bypass Graft	56,000	12,900	13,250	7,000
Pacemaker		7,500	5,000	3,500
Liposuction		5,000	2,133	2.500

The primary services being delivered by the exporting facilities and clinics can range widely and can include: Cardiac surgery including angioplasty, valve replacement and bypass surgery; orthopedic surgery including knee replacement, joints, hips, shoulder and spine; plastic and cosmetic surgery; dental implants, crowns and bridgework; bariatric and other weight loss surgery; infertility services; and spas which integrate yoga or Ayuravedic medicine and traditional Chinese medicine including acupuncture and other therapies. Some of these are more likely to be integrated with a vacation than others.

Particular countries have served different markets from abroad. Among the ASEAN nations Malaysia, Singapore and Thailand have made a concerted effort to attract patients from abroad as increasingly has the Philippines. Arunanondchail and Fink point out that the majority of patients in the recent past that visited Singapore and Malaysia came from other ASEAN countries but that in Thailand only seven percent of visitors were from other ASEAN countries while Japan was the leading source country but the US and the Middle East provided a number of patients as well. Mexico primarily attracts patients from the United States, both of Mexican origin as well as those born in the US. South Africa serves much of Southern Africa and Jordon has in recent years has been a leading exporter of services in the Middle East. Turkey in addition to attracting Turks who live in Europe seems well situated to attract patients from the former Soviet republics to its east and north as well as some from the Middle East. Regional centers of excellence can also attract patients from nearby countries who are seeking higher quality care than they believe they can obtain at home. Chile attracts many patients from Bolivia,

Tunisia serves many from Libya. And the US attracts many from Latin America and elsewhere. On the other hand a limited number of hospitals in Mexico seem to provide a high number of bariatric and other obesity related surgeries to uninsured and underinsured residents of Texas and nearby states .

Of advanced countries the US has both the largest number of uninsured —45 million —and underinsured and also the highest medical prices of any developed nation. This means that if someone has no coverage and limited means that they might be able to scrape up the cost of a hip resurfacing or knee operation abroad but it is not within their means in the US. Similarly even those with insurance in the US and elsewhere may find that operations they consider vital such as plastic or cosmetic surgery, bariatric surgery, or sex change operations may not be covered and only affordable if they go abroad. The potential market is constrained by the fact that for many who are uninsured or underinsured the out of pocket cost would still be severely difficult to meet. The economics are similar in countries where there are long waiting lists for elective procedures such as knee replacements or arthroscopic surgery and the individual has the means to purchase relief by going abroad.

Another category is patients who go overseas to obtain services for which they are eligible in their country of residence but for which the length of time they have to wait is significant. And it is possible that the service or procedure might not be available in time. One such procedure would be an organ transplant—especially a kidney or liver transplant. It is hard to know how many kidney transplants are done for international travelers and whether they have paid the donors for the kidneys. Over time a number of different arrangements have developed in different countries. Shimazono, who identified Pakistan, Iran, India, China and the Philippines as sources for commercial transplants, estimated that as much as 5% of the roughly 66,000 kidney transplants in 2005 worldwide were commercial transplants given to persons who travelled overseas . Merion and colleagues identified 373 foreign transplants from removals from waiting lists in the US between 2001 and 2006 due to having received a transplant from outside the US register. They believe that this was a minimum estimate and point out that the numbers of such removals increased between 2001 and 2006. Canales and associates identified 10 patients who were resident in Minnesota between 2002 and 2006 who received overseas transplants and returned to their kidney program in Minneapolis. They reported that the results were quite good. Eight were transplanted in Pakistan, one in China and one in Iran. There also seem to be a certain number of nonresidents who receive cadaver livers in the United States who have made major donations to the public or nonprofit transplant centers.

Also in the category of travelling to find services when they are not available in your own nation is the range of therapies categorized under the rubric of stem cell services. There has been a rapid proliferation of clinics which may make unsubstantiated and overly optimistic claims on their websites regarding the conditions for which stem cell therapy is appropriate and understating the possible negative side effects. Lau et al examined 19 websites of stem cell clinics located in India, Philippines, Russia, Mexico, China, Thailand, Turkey, Barbados, the Dominican Republic, and Ukraine. It is unclear how many people travel from abroad for these treatments—for the four sites that gave prices the cost averaged $21,000 excluding travel and lodging. The International Society for Stem Cell Research has issued new guidelines regarding core principles to guide the "transition of basic stem cell research into appropriate clinical applications."

Similarly there has been an increase in the numbers of persons who go abroad to fertility clinics, to find surrogate mothers at lower cost, or to have sex change operations. And a certain number of people go abroad for abortion services both for privacy and also in some cases because they are not legal in their nation of residence.

Tourists who Incidentally Need Care Abroad

Tourists and business travelers have been growing in numbers as the world has become more interdependent and as more and more people become able to afford such travel. Bookman and Bookman cite a study based on interviews with 17,000 travelers from 1996 to 2004 that showed that "eight percent of travelers to developing countries require medical care when on their trip (or immediately after). Usually it is for the treatment of diarrhea, although for travelers to Africa, the primary reason is malaria." Although most of this treatment is simply a doctor's visit and a prescription those who become more seriously in need of medical treatment either due to an accident or an acute event or due to a need for regular treatment for a chronic condition (such as dialysis) the availability of modern medical facilities makes traveling to or doing business in another country far more attractive.

Many travelers have insurance coverage for emergent conditions when they are on trips abroad. As the population in Japan and the West ages there will be more and more retirees going on extended trips to emerging countries and the availability of first class medical facilities will not only help to make many areas of the world more tourist friendly they may find more than historical levels of demand from this population.

Retirees Abroad

Finally, a group that is often not included in the category of medical tourists is retirees abroad. There are two distinct populations who retire abroad. One is people who are retiring to a country that they were not born in and have not been permanent residents in. This population may be seeking better climate, an interesting living arrangement, or lower costs in retirement. Since they often do not have health coverage when they retire abroad they may return to their country of prior residence when they need health services, but they are not usually considered to be medical tourists when they consume services in either country. The second population is persons who in retirement return to their country of origin. Although they are often entitled to health benefits in the country where they worked for many years such benefits may not be portable or only partially, so they also will return to their country of benefits for services or at least to a country where there is reciprocity for medical services. These trips back to the country where the benefits are also rarely qualifies as medical tourism.

It is very difficult to know how many people retire to a country different from the one where they have benefits. For those who are not returning to their native country it is often unclear whether they live part time in their new country or are permanent residents. For those who have returned to their native land they are often still citizens and captured as such both by the census and when they use facilities such as hospitals. If it is the case that roughly 200 million persons live in countries other than their country of birth it is not unreasonable to think that a significant number have also returned to their native land with entitlement to benefits in their nation of employment. Similarly there are probably even greater numbers of persons who have retired abroad. The reason this population is so important is that to the extent they are retiring from developed countries with comprehensive benefits they would cost the social insurance system a great deal if they remain. If they move to a lower cost developing nation they could receive health benefits at first class facilities and still cost the country in which they have benefits quite a lot less. In the US for instance where the total health expenditure per person was $7,421 in 2007 the expenditures on and by the over 65 population are substantially more per capita. Lack of portability probably means that many who would otherwise retire abroad do not.

INSURANCE COVERAGE

Each group who uses services abroad tends to have a different likelihood that they will have third party coverage for their care and different requirements to qualify for such coverage. Because this varies also by sending country and region it is worth reviewing this in some detail for travelers, for cross border plans, for people who buy such coverage directly and the kinds of employment or social insurance coverage that would permit or encourage such use.

Travellers Require Acute or Emergency Care

Travelers who incidentally have an acute or emergency need for medical coverage often are covered directly by their home insurance arrangements, by supplemental insurance they purchase or by the social welfare scheme of the country they find themselves in. In the EU travelers who have benefits in their home country have the EU health card or the E111 form and they are entitled to acute or emergency care in any other EU country. The benefit plans in some of the countries that reimburse for services received have developed networks of providers in other countries where many of their beneficiaries visit. Otherwise the beneficiary has to go to the public hospitals and clinics. Generally the invoices for care are aggregated at the national level and then reconciled at the EU level.

There has been some problem in making these reconciliations both because in Spain, for example, public hospitals may not aggregate these charges or compile or even collect them in a way so that the national authorities can make the case for their costs. At the EU level determining how to make the reconciliations between countries has been further compounded by countries that have a national health service and do not bill at point of service as compared to those where all patients are billed and their insurer pays. So not only is a bill not generated it is difficult to know what the appropriate price might be. This is compounded by the fact that in Britain a number of people have private coverage in addition to their national health coverage. Because of this complexity the National Health Service and individual EU countries with whom there is a great deal of travel have worked out aggregate annual payments to reconcile these accounts.

Between the EU and non EU countries reciprocity for such travelers is negotiated on an individual bilateral basis. For instance Britain has a reciprocity agreement to cover travelers with Australia, New Zealand, Malta, and some West Indian countries. Spain similarly has entered into agreements with Brazil, Chile, Ecuador, Peru and Paraguay as well as Andorra. Turkey has fairly extensive agreements with several EU countries. Other countries such as France and Germany have other bilateral arrangements.

In Canada most provinces have specific regulations that cover residents of the province when they are temporarily in another province or when they are outside the country. Generally if someone is a permanent resident of a province they will have some level of coverage when travelling outside the country. The length of time they can be out of the province will be generally from 6 months to 12 months if they are on vacation. Students, missionaries and certain categories of employees can be out of the country for a longer period. Each province also generally has limits on what they will pay for. The total amount spent in 2006—2007 for services outside the country for provinces that reported such figures ranged from $130,000 in Newfoundland and Labrador to $25 million in Ontario for out of country emergency inpatient and outpatient insured hospital and medical services. In that same year Ontario also spent $70.1 million for prior approved treatment outside Canada These figures do not include out of pocket expenditures or payments by private health insurance purchased by Canadians for care outside of Canada. Unlike in Britain where a number of persons buy private health insurance for care inside the country, in Canada such coverage is not available. But supplemental coverage is available for care or excess charges for care outside Canada.

In the US Medicare and Medicaid do not cover care outside the United States even for acute and emergency care while traveling unless it is on a direct trip between the lower 48 and Alaska or the facility is the closest appropriate facility for a medical incident that occurs inside the US. A fairly high number of people with Medicare coverage either have Medigap insurance that covers out of country acute and emergency care if it is during a trip of less than 60 days duration or they have a Medicare Advantage plan which offers comparable coverage. The 60 day limitation was established when Congress limited private insurers to 12 standard Medigap policies with clearly defined benefits so customers could make price comparisons. For the 10 standard policies that provide foreign coverage "....these policies pay for 80% of billed charges for certain medically necessary emergency care. The care is covered if it begins during the first 60 days of the trip, and if it isn't otherwise covered by Medicare. Foreign travel emergency coverage with Medicare policies has a lifetime limit of $50,000." Others may have an employee retirement benefit that provides such coverage beyond Medicare. Similarly many private policies by which the majority of people in the US are covered who are not covered by the government plans include coverage for emergency care abroad during a trip of limited duration from the United States. In addition a limited number of US citizens may have a Travel Medical Protection plan in addition to all this which covers evacuation as well as any bills uncovered by primary and secondary plans. The American Express plan covers care for the first 31 days of a covered trip up to $50,000 in uncovered expenses including evacuation. These plans generally do not cover pre existing conditions.

Cross Border Plans

Cross border plans can include plans that cover care in a border area, care to accommodate a large number of migrant workers from a contiguous nation, and care in an immigrant workers native land. In Europe there have been attempts to develop coverage in the border region between Belgium, Germany and the Netherlands so that economies of scale might be developed and also Belgium hospitals have entered into several contracts with British and Dutch Health authorities to provide care for persons with specific needs motivated in part by waiting lists at home.

In the United States several innovative plans have developed in California in which an employer offers a plan in which the employee, for a lower premium or little self pay, can choose to only receive their care at stipulated providers in Mexico. One of the plans, Access Baja, provides dual choice to groups of 50 or less so that employees can pick a Mexico only plan or the US plan. Salud con Healthnet is another plan which provides a network of providers in Los Angeles and Tijuana and enrollees can pick different provider options. For the Mexico part of its plan, Salud con Healthnet depends on Simnsa which runs two clinics and has contracts with hospitals in Tijuana. Simnsa also provides a plan in San Diego as well for care exclusively in Tijuana except for emergencies and services not available in Mexico.

The Western Growers Association provides a plan for its members which for a modest premium provides access to clinics and hospitals on the Mexican border to agricultural workers and their families. This plan covers an estimated 90,000 workers. Nearly all the workers who choose these plans are of Mexican origin and many have families in Mexico. One of the great deficiencies of the US health system is the large number of immigrants who are uninsured. In 2007, while 15.2% of the white 18-65 population of the US was uninsured, 59.3% of the Mexican immigrant population 18-65 was uninsured. Although these plans which are limited to care in Mexico are less expensive it is still hard to find employers willing to offer them and individuals are generally not willing to pay for them out of pocket.

Mexico in the past has offered their citizens in the United States the opportunity to buy themselves and their family members into the Mexican Social Security Program[IMSS]; but difficulty in processing the applications, cost, and limited availability of the IMSS in rural areas all have helped historically to keep enrollment in this program under 20,000. More recently the Mexican Secretary of Health has surfaced a proposal to help provide care for legal migrants and their families in Mexico in addition to access to care at Community Health Centers in the US which will be funded in part by migrants or their employers in the US.

Coverage for Medical Care Abroad

There has historically been health insurance for expatriate businesspeople and their families and some insurance that has targeted affluent persons in certain regions of the world; but the existence of insurance coverage that will cover elective care abroad is quite limited. Leading companies covering care for persons living abroad include Aetna Global benefits, United Health International, Blue Cross Blue Shield of America and BlueWorldwide Expat, CIGNA international, QBE in Australia, Goodhealth an Aetna company located in the UK and Bupa international in the UK. Aetna Global Benefits "is the international health and group benefits business of Aetna Inc., one of the world's leading providers of health and group benefits. [It]....currently provides coverage for more than 100,000 expatriate and other international employees residing and/or traveling in over 100 countries. Aetna Global Benefits products are tailored to meet the unique needs of global members, providing worldwide medical, dental, life, disability and related coverage that helps multinational employers attract and retain qualified employees for overseas assignments." Most of the other firms would describe their mission similarly and in many cases not only have developed networks of providers worldwide but are also geared up to pay for care back in the home country.

British United Provident Associates (BUPA) acquired both Amedex and International Health Insurance Danmark in recent years. In addition to its international health insurance business for travelers and expatriates Bupa international has continued the Amedex line of business which covered mostly affluent residents of Latin America and the Caribbean for care anywhere in the Western hemisphere in many of their products. David Maltby says, "Many Latin Americans often travel overseas for medical treatment which is why we have designed our new products to fit with people's different lifestyles and health requirements....there is a policy to meet your needs and those of your family." Similarlly the Azul or premium versions of policies written by Grupo Nacional Provincial in Mexico have covered care in the US as well as in Mexico. In both cases the more expensive policies provide subscribers coverage for care in other nations.

The EU has recently clarified the rights of citizens of its member countries to choose to seek nonemergency care in other countries in the EU. This was the consequence of several decisions by the European Court of Justice and the result of extensive deliberations amongst the countries of the EU. The proposed directive, which will be considered by the European Parliament and the Council of Ministers in the coming months, establishes that patients may seek ambulatory care abroad for any services they are entitled to in their own country and to be reimbursed for their costs up to the level of reimbursement in their own country. The directive also establishes a right to hospital care and treatment abroad up to the level the patient is entitled to in their own country but it does say that "under certain circumstances a Member state may decide to introduce a system in which patients require an administrative prior authorization before seeking care abroad.". A number of safeguards, including equal treatment of those who seek care abroad, availability of patient records, recognition of pharmaceuticals needed in continuity of treatment, and legal recourse for medical errors, are also built into the directive. There is nothing in the directive that implies it could be extended to other countries as well. At the same time one might think that natives of Turkey, Algeria, or India or Pakistan who are entitled to these benefits might not have at least a moral case that they should be able to return "home" for care and be reimbursed on the same basis.

In the United States the large number of uninsured persons as well as many with limited coverage or with large deductibles or some with Medical savings accounts has led to estimates that there is likely to be a substantial market for international coverage in the future. Although in principle it would be possible to incentivize such care by covering travel costs and preferential cost sharing for those who travel to preferred providers in practice it has been difficult. Health insurance in the United States is generally regulated by the state in which the person lives. But, if the employer "self insures"—bearing some of the risk, then they escape regulation by the states and can develop more innovative benefit plans. In general there seems to be reluctance by insurers to develop plans that would force beneficiaries into going to foreign providers since they could be considered liable if there are bad results and they might be considered the one deep pocket.

Individuals who are uninsured or not insured for something like plastic surgery or bariatric surgery have been the most likely to choose to travel long distances. This is for two reasons; on the one hand if they are uninsured they often have to pay the retail rate which is often more than twice as much as the rate commercial insurers are able to negotiate or government programs like Medicare of Medicaid pay. The second reason is that they often have a very specific need such as chronic hip pain, or a desire for plastic or bariatric surgery and they are able to come up with the specific funds needed to pay for the trip abroad and the care. Given their limited resources the only choice is whether they want to do the procedure abroad or not at all. In fact there is a Canadian firm [North American Surgery] which specializes in finding US providers who will take less for many of these procedures and that seems to skim off some of those from the US or Canada who would consider going abroad. With increased unemployment there will certainly be more in the US who are uninsured; but at the same time with economic uncertainty people may be less likely to spend funds on discretionary medical procedures.

And part of the Obama stimulation package that has passed the house but not the Senate is a temporary subsidy for persons who have lost their jobs to be able to continue their health insurance coverage. In 2008, "3 percent of the population was enrolled in a consumer-driven health plan [DCHP], up from 2 per cent in 2007 and 1 percent in 2006. Enrollment in HDHPs remained at 11 percent. Overall, 9.8 million adults ages 21-64 with private insurance (representing 6.6 percent of that market) were either in a CDHP or an HDHP that was eligible for an HAS [Health Savings Account], but had not opened the account.". Although high deductible plans do encourage savings and cost effective medical use the cost of surgery overseas would tend to exceed the deductible in any case so that the net savings to the individual is likely to be negligible.

There are a number of pilot programs that have been inaugurated for coverage overseas but there is limited evidence since their launch. Aetna initiated a program for Hannaford Supermarkets where Aetna offered to cover certain procedures outside the United States. "Workers go to Singapore for hip replacement surgery without incurring any out-of-pocket medical costs. In addition the patient and a companion get free airfare and hotel accommodations." Aetna reports that "a plan member would save about $3,000 by going to Singapore." As of June 2008, "not one of Hannaford's 27,000 workers has selected the foreign care option, not have any other large-employee groups asked Aetna to include it as an option, according to a spokesman for the insurer.".

Blue Cross Blue Shield of South Carolina has spun off Companion Global Health Care as an independent subsidiary. The subsidiary has offered a medical tourism option to Doctors Care who operate health clinics. To date none of the 1000 employees and dependents covered by Doctors Care have chosen to go abroad since the option has been available. Wellpoint [which is the agglomeration of former Blue Cross Blue Shield plans that are for profit] is starting a similar program beginning in January 2009 through its affiliate Anthem of Wisconsin. They are providing access to a network of providers in India at a reduced out of pocket costs to employees of Serigraph—a Wisconsin based provider of printed decorating solutions.

A somewhat different approach is that taken by Sekure Health Plans which has developed a network of providers in the US and throughout Mexico who have negotiated prices for services. Services include diet counseling, massage therapy, chiropractic and acupuncture in addition to standard medical and dental services. A group or individual can purchase membership which entitles them to these prices if they use a network provider. Portions of the network can be used in conjunction with a limited benefit medical insurance plan. A similar model might be developed with a wider package of international providers in the network. Swiss Re has developed the option of medical care abroad for self funded employers in the US who purchase their stop loss coverage. In principal there should not be a difficulty including selected hospitals and clinics abroad in a PPO so long as the plan is self insured.

Portability of Coverage in Retirement

There are two distinct populations who wish to retire abroad and, for both, portability of the health benefits they are entitled to so that their care will be covered in the country they choose to retire to can make a major difference in whether or not they choose to retire abroad and the burden they may impose on the country they retire to. The first population includes persons who choose to retire abroad from their native country because of cost, amenities, cultural interest, or a desire to be of service. The second population includes those who wish to return to their native country in retirement. There are some differences between these two groups and also some differences in entitlements and portability so we will discuss them separately.

It is also important to note that the population entering their retirement years will grow very rapidly over the next decades in many countries. In the US in 2006 there were 31.6 million persons 55-64, 18.9 million 65-74, 13.2 million 75-84 and 5 million 85 and over. In Europe in 2007 in France, Germany, Italy and Great Britain alone there were more than 45 million persons 65 and over. In Japan there were more than 26.8 million over 65 in 2007. And in China while there were 102 million persons 65 and over in 2007 there will be an estimated 322 million by 2050.All of these countries not only will have a growing portion of their population entering these ages they all face serious fiscal challenges to find a way to support this population and provide health care as well.

Many currently do choose to retire abroad. Large numbers of northern Europeans retire to Spain, Portugal, Greece and Italy. Retirees from the US and Canada are increasingly retiring to Mexico, Costa Rica, Panama, and even Ecuador. Retirement communities are springing up and expanding in several locations in Baja California, along the Mexican Pacific coast, the gulf of Cortez and in Yucatan for example. Japan also has in the past considered the development of Silver towns where retirees could more economically retire. The attraction is the climate, much lower expenses, very low property taxes and the ability to hire household help at affordable rates. But for many the lack of medical coverage when abroad can make it difficult to remain abroad in retirement or deters them from considering the option in the first place.

In the EU as discussed above retirees can move their entitlement from one country to another country in the EU. If they are moving from the UK to Spain for instance it means that they then use the Spanish public system and need to move their coverage back to the UK if they decide to return. Many retirees instead use their EU health card as if they are temporarily abroad when they have an acute incident or an emergency and then pay out of pocket for routine care and return home for more serious needs. Alternatively some of the health insurance schemes in Germany and elsewhere have developed networks of providers where tourists and retirees are likely to be so it is not necessary to transfer ones coverage. At the same time many who are dependent on the state for financial assistance are not able to continue to receive that if they leave their home country. Coverage outside the EU only is available through bilateral agreements.

In the US some retirees abroad have coverage through their corporate retirement coverage although that often will not cover care for extended care abroad. Since 2000, Tricare, which is the health coverage for military retirees and their dependents, covers care for beneficiaries living abroad. The Veterans Administration will cover care for service connected disabilities. The vast majority, however, do not have coverage after the age of 65 except through Medicare and Medigap policies which will not cover care for those residing abroad.

Medicare Part B [physician and outpatient diagnostic] coverage and $30 or more a month for Medicare prescription coverage even though neither will pay for care or drugs obtained in Mexico. If a beneficiary does not continue this coverage [the premiums are subtracted from Social Security checks] then they have to wait to be reinstated and for every year they are not covered their future Part B premiums increase by 10 per cent a year and their drug premiums by one percent a month.

It would appear clear that if Medicare coverage were available to retirees to Mexico that more would retire there, that the costs to Medicare might be significantly less, and that future social service and Medicaid costs in nursing homes might be averted to the extent that people would be able to stay in their homes and to pay for assistance in Mexico. The Mexican government requested in the annual meeting of NAFTA finance ministers in August of 2007 that such coverage be provided. Both the Philippines and Panama have made a similar request. In all cases it was suggested that the Center for Medicare and Medicaid Services [CMS] be authorized to conduct a pilot study of making such coverage portable or possibly grant a waiver so retirees to these countries would be covered. In the 2008 election the Democrats Abroad advocated that Medicare coverage for retirees abroad should be implemented. So far CMS has stated that it requires Congress to authorize any international demonstration program. It would seem to be prudent for CMS to at least do some test experiments to see what the cost, access and quality of care issues might be in serving a population that is only likely to get much larger.

For those who wish to return to their native land after many years abroad the ability to bring the capacity to pay for first class health services would not only make the transition more attractive for the individual, it would also make the individual a more significant financial asset to the original sending country. In all cases this might not be necessary. Greece and Australia concluded a social security treaty in which workers were entitled to combine years worked in both systems for the determination of their social security benefits and for those who returned to Greece who had had at least one year working in the Greek Social Insurance system the pensioner and his family are entitled to healthcare coverage under the Greek system. There are large numbers of immigrant workers in Europe, North America, the Gulf, and Japan, Hong Kong, and Australia. Europe has concluded some agreements on coordination of pensions with Algeria, Morocco, and Tunisia and Turkey has extensive agreements as well. Portability of health benefits in retirement seems to be an issue which needs to be negotiated on a bilateral basis between the two nations. Turkey seems to have negotiated an agreement whereby a retiree back to Turkey who has worked substantially their working career in Germany or Austria or the Netherlands or indeed other nations in the EU has portable benefits back in Turkey from the country where they worked. Morocco has negotiated a similar arrangement with Germany. Morocco's arrangement with Austria however just stipulates that Austria will pay no more in Morocco than it would pay as a charge in Austria; but Austria's hospitals are heavily subsidized and the charges are consequently well below cost. Austria will pay a Turkish retiree up to full Austrian cost since that is what is stipulated in their agreement. On the other hand a Moroccan who receives a French pension and returns to Morocco has a monthly contribution to the French public health system taken out of their pension but has not access to care in Morocco.

Most of the states in the Gulf do not permit migrants to become citizens but they do encourage them to buy into retirement schemes in their home countries. And generally it seems they are expected to fend for themselves back in their home countries at the end of their term[s] in the Gulf. In Asia the Philippines is a major exporting country—most who go to Japan or Saudi Arabia return to the Philippines in retirement.

In the US Mexican immigrants who work the equivalent of 10 years are eligible to retire at 62 under Social Security and to receive Medicare at 65. If they are undocumented than they may find it very difficult to claim these earned benefits. However Medicare will not cover services for them when they return home in any case. There are also a number of Mexican immigrants to the US who are permanent residents but who never became citizens primarily because of limited English proficiency. Such persons are not allowed to leave the US for more than six months at a time. Thus even if they had portable

Medicare coverage and could in principle retire to Mexico they would have to make sure that they never stayed longer than six months at a time. Otherwise they could lose their permanent resident status and also their rights to Medicare.

It is hard to know how many migrants to the wealthier states are likely to return to their native country—estimates based on experiences in the 19th and first half of the 20th Centuries seem to imply quite a wide range. In any case it would not be unusual to think that fairly soon there would be at least 25-30 million who have returned if not all of retirement age. That combined with 3-5 million retirees from Europe, North America, Japan, and elsewhere, who have decided to retire to nations such as Mexico, Costa Rica, the Philippines, Malaysia, Panama, India, north Africa, Fiji, Tahiti, Brazil, Turkey, and Argentina could mean a major possible infusion of funds into these countries both for medical care and to support the economy. One million persons spending $10,000 per capita on living and $5,000 on average on medical care can bring $15 billion annually in foreign exchange into an economy. There is also some developing interest in the Doha round to take the position that such immigrants as Mode 4 workers are entitled to the same benefits in retirement as those native workers they worked alongside.

Increased globalization will certainly lead to increased cross border utilization of services. Because of an ingrained preference for receiving care in ones country of residence it is unlikely that even with coverage for medical tourism that all of the "economic advantage" will be achieved by covering such care—in part because the person covered is unlikely to reap many of the benefits. It does appear that substantial benefits would arise for all concerned if health coverage in retirement could follow retirees to the countries where they retire. Countries can continue to address some of these issues on a bilateral basis but a broader perspective might be warranted. Although Joint Commission Certification is a good first step towards determining quality it might be a good idea to develop mandatory reporting of medical errors and infection rates not only at "exporting hospitals and clinics" but also at hospitals and clinics in the US, Japan and Europe. Similarly some method of certifying web sites and their claims both for those maintained by providers and independent ones should be undertaken.

Perhaps more objective audits need to be developed so that quality, cost, and possible problems can be better identified and made public.

At this point there does not seem to be much movement by nations under the GATS to open up the private or public health insurance markets in the sense of requiring that insurers cover care abroad as if it took place in their home country. The GATS is not an impediment to a country deciding to tax their first class hospitals which are serving medical tourists. This is an export industry and a nation can tax its exports freely. Even with an agreement by insurers not to discriminate between foreign and domestic providers it is hard to see why travel costs would need to be covered.

In some ways the EU is developing protocols within the EU whereby citizens can receive care across national boundaries. Perhaps as the EU better develops protocols and arrangements with countries outside the EU, Japan and the US will begin to do so as well. Further study is required to evaluate and develop insurance initiatives both in the private sector and the public sector as well.

Medical Tourism: Trends in Asia

Medical tourism has grown in a number of countries, such as India, Singapore and Thailand, many of which have deliberately linked medical care to tourism, and thus boost the attractions of nearby beaches etc. But medical tourism has also developed in South Africa and in countries not hitherto associated with significant levels of western tourism such as Belarus, Latvia, Lithuania and Costa Rica. Hungary, for example, declared 2003 to be the Year of Health Tourism. Eastern European countries have become important for dental care and plastic surgery. Jordan serves patients from some parts of the Middle East while Israel caters both to Jewish patients and others from nearby countries, through specialising in female infertility, in vitro fertilisation and high-risk pregnancies.

South Africa has grown in prominence in recent years, especially for cosmetic surgery, since its costs are less than half those of the United States, from where most of its patients come. Argentina is also noted for plastic surgery. The Caribbean has found it more difficult to enter the medical tourism market since, despite its proximity to the United States, its prices cannot compete with those in Latin America.

Some Caribbean states have sought to get around this by specialisation, hence Cuba specialises in skin diseases and Antigua in dentistry. In the Pacific Guam has become a regional dental centre for Palau, the Federated States of Micronesia and also Japan.

As one of the main sources of medical tourists, the Middle East—particularly Dubai, but also Bahrain and Lebanon—has recently sought to reverse this flow and develop its own medical tourism industry. Dubai has just built Healthcare City (DHCC) to capture the Middle Eastern market and try and divert it from Asia. Unable to compete on price the Middle East has largely competed on quality, with Dubai bringing in German doctors to guarantee high skill standards, and Lebanon stressing its many doctors trained in Europe and America. Branding is seen as important; 'it remains to be seen if DHCC will attract peopley if there is a single hospital that had one or two good brands that would be good if there was a Cleveland Clinic or a Guy's or Thomas's Hospital'. Saudi Arabia has sought to link medical tourism, and especially cosmetic surgery and dentistry, with pilgrimage (Hajj) visits to the country, with most patients being from other Gulf countries, and the Health Minister of Iran has claimed that 'No Middle East country can compete with Iran in terms of medical expertise and costs', comparing the cost of open heart surgery at US$18,000 in Turkey, $40,000 in UK and $10,000 in Iran so that patients 'can afford the rest on touring the country'. In 2005 relatively low cost Jordan remained the main medical tourism destination in the Middle East.

As medical tourism has grown in Asia rich world countries have also sought involvement. Thus the Bavaria Medical Group (BMG) has developed links with Qatar Airways and the Sultanate of Oman that have taken patients from Oman to Germany and also resulted in specialist BMG doctors visiting Oman. However, rich countries can rarely compete, and restore the old order, as medical tourism has reversed direction. In a very short time period the global structure of health tourism has become highly complex.

The main region for medical tourism is Asia. Thailand became known as a destination for medical tourism as early as the 1970s because it specialised in sex change operations, and later moved into cosmetic surgery. Malaysia became involved after 1998 in the wake of the Asian economic crisis and the need for economic diversification, as did many Thai hospitals, when local patients were no longer able to afford private health care. Singapore has belatedly sought to compete with Malaysia and Thailand, deliberately set rates just below those in Thailand and even set up a stand at the airport with fliers, information and advice for transit passengers.

India is usually regarded as the contemporary global centre for medical tourism, and it advertises itself as offering everything from alternative Ayurvedic therapy to coronary bypasses and cosmetic surgery. To become the most important global destination it has upgraded technology, absorbed western medical protocols and emphasised low cost and prompt attention. Since economic liberalisation in the mid-1990s private hospitals have expanded and found it easier to import technology and other medical goods, thus bringing infrastructure in the best hospitals to western levels. The links to India's highly successful IT industry are also advertised as important. Moreover, as hospitals improved and specific salaries increased, so doctors returned from overseas. Many had international qualifications and western experience that could be advertised to make potential tourists more comfortable.

The same liberalisation brought new structures of corporatisation that streamlined India's notorious bureaucracy and significantly improved administration. The principal corporate hospital chains employ teams of interpreters, though India has benefited because of its widespread English speaking ability. While technology has become much the same as in the west, and doctors are experienced in western procedures, most labour costs remain very low and insurance is less costly. Success rates, even for procedures that can have high infection rates, such as heart operations, bone marrow transplants and kidney transplants, are comparable to those at some of the world's best hospitals. India has an annual Medical Tourism Expo and it has been predicted that medical tourism will earn India as much as US$2 billion by 2012.

Measures of the flows of medical tourists vary enormously, partly because this defies easy categorisation (either in terms of patients and/or accompanying family members etc.) and partly because no statistics distinguish it. The only specific survey undertaken appears to have been in Costa Rica where a 1991 university study found that 14 percent of all visitors to Costa Rica came to receive some sort of medical care, usually cosmetic surgery and dental work . In terms of origin it has been estimated that about 50,000 people left the UK in 2003 as medical tourists. Thailand claims to have the largest number of medical tourists, with a million patients from Japan in 2003 and a 20 percent increase in 2004, and has been credited by Singapore with having 800,000 overseas patients in 2003 but there are no reliable data to demonstrate this. It has also been reported that in 2004 some 247,238 Japanese, 118,701 American, 95,941 UK and 35,092 Australian patients were treated in Thai hospitals, though this includes locally based expatriates and other injured and sick tourists. One estimate for India was of 150,000 medical tourists visiting in 2002, almost half of whom came from the Middle East, but it has been estimated that the number will reach about 500,000 in 2005. Another recent estimate for 2004 put the annual inflow to India between 10,000 and 20,000 foreign patients and another repeated the 150,000 figure. At the end of the last century the number of foreign patients seeking medical treatment in Malaysia was estimated to have been around 400,000 over a two-year period; this is likely to be an overestimate, as some 150,000 were reported in 2004. Singapore claimed an annual 150,000 international patients in 2003, was reported as having 230,000 foreigners seeking medical care in 2003 and was recently said to have an annual 200,000 medical tourists. Certainly numbers are steadily rising in most destinations, but there are no reliable national figures for any country.

Economic Benefits

Medical tourists not surprisingly are mainly from rich world countries where the costs of medical care may be very high, but where the ability to pay for alternatives is also high. Most are from North America, Western Europe and the Middle East. In India a majority are part of the Indian Diaspora in the United States, Britain and elsewhere, but include elites from a range of countries, including several African states, but there has been a gradual shift to a more diverse patient population. One Chennai (Madras) hospital has claimed patients from Oman, UAE, Bahrain, Qatar, Saudi Arabia, Mauritius, Seychelles, Maldives, Sri Lanka, Bhutan, Nepal, East Africa, Germany, Australia, Canada and the UK.

European patients favour India, Thailand and Malaysia. Early on, Malaysia primarily focused on the Middle East, stressing its Islamic credentials, including the presence of halal food and Islamic practices in hospitals. The manager of one group of Malaysian hospitals has said 'since 9/11 people started looking to the Eastern world for holidays and we are trying to capture a fraction of these people. The Middle East is a huge market for us. Abu Dhabi Company for Onshore Oil Operations sends its 36,000 employees to us for checkups. Since 9/11 Thailand has gained contracts from the UAE's police department and the Oman Government, both of which were formerly linked to Europe. Malaysia has also organised trade missions to such south east Asian countries as Myanmar and Vietnam, where there is a small potential elite market, and it receives a large number of medical visitors from Indonesia. However, 70 percent of those people from UAE who travel overseas for health treatment are said to go to Singapore and India is said to be the preferred destination of Omanis. Many patients in both Malaysia and Singapore are Europeans and Americans resident in Asia. Singapore has seen a shift of its market from Indonesia to the Middle East, alongside ethnic Chinese from a diversity of sources. Rich Japanese tend to fly to Singapore, and Sumatrans go by ferry to Malaysia. Thailand has deliberately sought a Japanese market, since many doctors have been trained in Japan, and nurses and other staff have been taught to speak Japanese; Thailand mainly has patients from Japan, Brunei, Singapore, Taiwan, Pakistan, China and Bangladesh. Cuba has a primarily Latin American market with Argentina, Ecuador and also the Dominican Republic as the main sources of medical tourists. The global migration of doctors, especially from India to Europe and North America has meant growing familiarity with being treated by Indians and Filipinos.

Japan has always been unwilling to accept immigration hence has a health care system that is under considerable pressure, especially as its population ages, without access to migrant health workers as in most other developed countries. Consequently Japan has taken particular advantage of the notion of medical tourism. Many Japanese companies even send their employees to Thailand and Singapore for annual physical examinations, as the savings on medical fees and high-quality medical care make the airfare inconsequential. For provincial Japanese companies the cost is little more that of travelling to Tokyo, reports are done in Japanese and images sent electronically to Japan. Moreover at least one Bangkok hospital has an exclusively Japanese wing and there are many Japanese nursing homes in Bangkok.

Economics effectively calibrates the rise of medical tourism. Price differentials between most Asian states and more developed countries are considerable and are presently diverging even further. This may be accentuated or influenced by long waiting lists. For complex surgery the differences are considerable. In 2003 a small child in the United States with a hole in her heart was faced with a bill of around $70,000 there, but the operation was carried out in Bangalore, India at a cost of $4400. Open heart surgery may cost about $70,000 in Britain and up to $150,000 in the United States but in India's best hospitals it costs between $3000 and $10,000 depending on how complicated it is. Dental, eye and cosmetic surgery costs about a quarter of that in western countries. The price differentials for cosmetic surgery are particularly significant since cosmetic procedures are not covered by insurance. A face-lift in Costa Rica costs about a third of that in the United States, and rather less in South Africa. However, any complications and postoperative costs may have to be met in the patient's home country, hence disparaging comments that this is 'fly in fly out' or 'itinerant surgery'. Patients in a sense are outsourcing themselves.

Currency fluctuations can be a significant influence. When the South African Rand rose significantly in value against the US dollar in 2004, one company went from about 30 patients a month in 2003 to none in 2005.

India has cornered a substantial part of the market because its fees are significantly below those of other possible destinations. Thus bypass operations in India are about a sixth of the cost in Malaysia. Nonetheless, price differentials between all Asian countries and the west remain considerable: Thailand can offer liposuction and breast enhancement surgery for a fifth of the rate this would cost in Germany, hence it has focused on this particular European market. Singapore has sought to compete on quality rather than price and stresses its superior technology, and that Singapore doctors had carried out the first Asian separation of Siamese twins and the first South East Asian heart transplant, amongst other similar 'firsts'.

While economic benefits are central to medical tourism they are not the only factors. Waiting lists for nonessential surgery such as knee reconstructions may be as long as 18 months in the UK. In India the whole procedure can be done in under a week and patients sent home after a further 10 days. Some surgery, such as this, regarded as nonessential or low priority in the western world, may be necessary for certain forms of employment, and hence worth travelling for. Similarly, in the UK, waiting times for fertility treatments may be very long, and at an important period in couples' lives, hence many 'fertility tourists' have gone overseas.

Distance offers anonymity. Some medical procedures, such as sex changes, have become small but significant parts of medical tourism, especially in Thailand, where recuperation and the consolidation of a new identity may be better experienced at a distance from standard daily life. Similarly cosmetic surgery patients may prefer recuperation in a relatively alien environment.

Even where privacy may not necessarily seem to be crucial to the operation, that it parallels exclusivity can be important. Thus the Mauritius hair grafting clinic, whose name suggests an elite Parisian connection, argues 'situated not far from most exclusive hotels, the clinic receives patients from around the world. Many stars and persons of international fame, who naturally require the utmost discretion, owe the restoration of their hair to this clinic'.

Distance also offers alternatives. Certain operations may not be available in origin countries. Abortions are banned in several countries or are restricted to early periods of pregnancy. In Britain, for example, health authorities are usually unwilling to countenance stomach stapling for patients if they are aged less than 18; this is not the case in many medical tourism destinations where the 'customer' is more likely to be right.

The most extreme forms of such travel, where the word tourism fits least easily, are those of patients seeking euthanasia. In recent years this has brought a stream of non-citizens to Switzerland, may have taken 'death tourists' to the Netherlands and for a time in the 1990s took Australians to the Northern Territory (the only part of the country where euthanasia was briefly permissible). A final form is a variant of 'transnational retirement': the establishment of overseas nursing homes, where patients effectively stay permanently, as in Kenya, where converted hotels (as the tourism market declines) have been turned into homes for east African Asians, retiring and returning from the UK, or for Japanese in Thailand and the Philippines.

Medical tourism is likely to increase even faster in the future as medical care continues to be increasingly privatised, and cost differentials remain in place. As the demand for cosmetic surgery (including dentistry) continues to expand so will demand for overseas services, and this will probably replace heart surgery as the core element in medical tourism. Moreover, as successful outcomes become more evident, demand is likely to increase further. Western insurance companies might encourage overseas treatment to reduce their own costs. The trade in health services is expanding, becoming more competitive, and creating new dimensions of globalisation, all elegantly packaged, and sometimes actually functioning, as the new niche of medical tourism.

References

Arunanondchai, Jutamas and Carson Fink, (2006)."Trade in Health Services in the ASEAN region," *Health Promotion International,* Vol. 21 pp. 59-66.

Bookman, Milica Z. and Karla R. Bookman, (2007).*Medical Tourism in Developing Countries*, Palgrave Macmillan, NY.

Canales, MT, BL Kasiske, ME Rosenberg, (2007)."Transplant Tourism: Outomes of United States Residents Who Undergo Transplantation Overseas," *Transplantation,* Vol 82, No. 12, 1858-1862.

Cortez, Nathan, (2008)."Patients Without Borders: The Emerging Global Market for Patients and the Evolution of Modern Health Care," *Indiana Law Journal*, Volume 83: pp. 71-132.

Lautier, Marc, (2008)."Export of Health Services from Developing Countries: The Case of Tunisia," Social Science and Medicine, 67, pp.101-110.

Woodman, Josef, (2008). *Patients Beyond Borders: Affordable World Class Medical Travel, Healthy Travel Media*, Chapel Hill, North Carolina.

3

Globalization of Healthcare Marketplace

In the last decade, and primarily in the present century the notion of well being has gone further than ever before. No longer is improved health on holiday merely an anticipated consequence of escape from the arduous drudgery of work and the movement to a place with a cleaner (or warmer) climate, or the outcome of 'taking the waters', but in some circumstances—the rise of medical tourism—it has become the central theme of tourism in an active rather than a passive sense. A new niche has emerged in the tourist industry. While some writers have continued to use the phrase 'health tourism' to cover all forms of health-related tourism, it seems more useful to distinguish 'medical tourism' as one involving specific medical interventions.

Medical tourism as a niche has emerged from the rapid growth of what has become an industry, where people travel often long distances to overseas countries to obtain medical, dental and surgical care while simultaneously being holidaymakers, in a more conventional sense. It has grown dramatically in recent years primarily because of the high costs of treatment in rich world countries, long waiting lists (for what is not always seen institutionally as priority surgery), the relative affordability of international air travel and favourable economic exchange rates, and the ageing of the often affluent postwar baby-boom generation. It has thus largely reversed an earlier pattern of wealthy patients travelling to rich world centres, such as Harley Street in London (but where tourism was not involved). Growth has been facilitated by the rise of the Internet, and the emergence of new companies, that are not health specialists, but brokers between international patients and hospital networks. It has also grown because of rapidly improving health care systems in some key countries, where new technologies have been adopted. Above all it has followed the deliberate marketing of health care (in association with tourism) as medical care has gradually moved away from the public sector to the private sector, ensuring that a growing majority of people, especially in the richest countries, and particularly in the United States, must pay often considerably for health care. Finally, growing interest in cosmetic surgery, involving such elective procedures as rhinoplasty, liposuction, breast enhancement or reduction, LASIK eye surgery and so on, or more simply the removal of tattoos, have created new demands. Various forms of dental surgery, especially cosmetic dental surgery, are not covered by insurance in countries like the UK and Australia; hence dental tourism has become particularly common. In Asia these trends are 'the unlikely child of new global realities: the fallout of terrorism, the Asian economic downturn, internet access to price information, and the globalisation of health services'.

The biggest hurdle that medical tourism has had to face, and continues to face, is the challenge of convincing distant potential visitors that medical care in relatively poor countries is comparable with that available at home, in outcome, safety and even in dealing with pain thresholds. This has been especially so when medical care systems, in countries such as India, have been conventionally regarded in the west as inadequate, 'even' for India itself. As the German radio station, Deutsche Welle, has pointed out 'India is not exactly known for health and hygiene' yet it nonetheless anticipates a major market in Germany. Attached to that is the parallel perception that 'you get what you pay for', hence cheap medical care may well be inferior. While such situations have now radically changed the perception of inadequacy remains.

Growth of Medical Tourism Industry

Medical tourism has a long history, but what is new is its unprecedented growth at the global level. The first known and documented medical tourists were ancient pilgrims who used to travel from all over the Mediterranean to Epidauria in the Saronic Gulf, a sanctuary of the healing God Asklepios, for treatment. Traditionally, the rich and the aristocrats travelled abroad, to the spa towns and sanitariums of their favourite medical destinations, for mineral baths, innovative therapies and fairer climates to improve their health. The recent trend in medical travel, however, is significantly different from these earlier ones and can best be described as travel from developed countries, by the middle class, to a foreign country to avoid treatment delays, to receive affordable, quality medical care or simply to have elective surgery combined with sightseeing and other local tourism opportunities.

It is not clearly known when and how the modern version of medical tourism saw its first real boom. It has been reported that the Asian financial crisis in 1997 led many Southeast Asian nations, particularly Thailand, to seek alternative strategies to cope with their emerging economies. As many private hospitals and health facilities lost their local affluent customer base due to the economic crisis, physicians and other health providers in Thailand began leaving their country to work elsewhere, while private hospitals were forced to change their marketing strategies and target patients from overseas for their survival.

The customers of modern medical tourism are primarily from rich countries such as the United States, Canada, Britain, Australia, the Middle East and Japan. Although Thailand, India, Singapore, Malaysia, Jordan and some countries in South America are currently the most popular choices among medical travellers, the industry has been growing rapidly in other parts of the world as well. The number of medical travellers has been difficult to estimate as no systematic data are recorded and the reported number of medical travellers may have included business travellers and regular tourists who needed medical care while they were abroad.

According to the most widely accepted estimate, nearly 350,000 patients from all industrialized nations travelled to a variety of less developed countries for health care in 2003. Since then the number of medical tourists has been increasing exponentially, particularly from the USA. In 2007, nearly 750,000 US patients travelled overseas for medical treatment, while the figure increased to nearly 1.5 million in 2008. It has been projected that the number of American medical travellers could reach 6 million by 2010 and more than 15 million by 2017.

The medical tourism industry used to provide cosmetic surgeries and dental procedures in earlier decades. Current medical travellers receive virtually all types of health care from cosmetic or dental care to knee or hip replacements, from cardiac and eye surgeries to organ transplants and surrogacy at medical facilities in developing countries.

Spending for the medical tourism business has been growing quickly as well. While no coordinated system is in place to gather and compile financial information for this sector, studies indicate that medical tourism worldwide could generate as much as $40 billion by 2010. One projection estimates that US patients alone will spend more than $40 billion for health care services abroad by 2017. Other estimates indicate that the worldwide revenue for medical tourism was about $60 billion in 2006, which could increase to $100 billion by 2012.

Although medical tourism has become a major sector in the global health care system, research has remained scarce. Not only is reliable and internationally comparable information on the number of travellers or the amount of money spent on travel unavailable, but the concepts and definitions that encompass medical tourism are not standardized.

The dominant theme remains: medical tourism growth is exclusively an outcome of recent crises in the provision of Western medical care including the relentless, decades-long rise in the cost of health care and non-responsiveness to the public's demand for timely care. The growth of medical tourism is viewed as a transient effect of such crises, with the added allure of adventure and vacation in countries far from home.

The impact of medical tourism on the health systems in provider countries has received a lot of attention in the literature. It has been viewed simultaneously as a blessing to the economy and as a threat to national health systems. Potential negative consequences include widening disparities due to unequal distribution of health care, financial deprivation of medical professionals who are delivering world class health services for third world prices, subsidizing costs of care for patients of rich countries, and diverting resources from the poor and disadvantaged to patients from abroad. Although logical in themselves, such claims are rarely articulated within theoretical premises that might offer explanations for how and to what extent the growth of medical tourism creates major risks for the health sector, or benefits to the economy, of provider countries.

The literature also focuses on concerns about the safety of patients travelling abroad to receive care and the accompanying risks of carrying infectious diseases back home from provider countries. Considerable emphasis has been given to potential violations of human rights through the practice of illicit activities that the medical tourism trade allegedly promotes, notably in medical transplantation, surrogacy and such aesthetic surgeries as abdominoplasty, rhinoplasty or bariatric surgery. These may be illegal or regarded as immoral in countries from which medical tourists originate but are allowed in provider countries. However, available literature has rarely focused on the failure of global initiatives to control illicit medical practices or the role of governments of the provider countries to prohibit transplant tourism.

Economic Impacts of Medical Tourism Business

The growth of medical tourism, as a new business model, cannot be explained without looking at its interactions with economic, social and political forces. Studies have attempted to link the determinants of its expansion with the demand and supply of health services in the context of changing and variant market prices across the globe. Globalization-led economic restructuring has created a space for investment in private sector health programs in many developing countries: to expand its health services to cater to patients from abroad and compete among themselves for the market. For the patients in developed countries where the cost of health care is very high or they have to wait for a long time to get treatment, this emerging market has provided wider choices to buy health services with variant prices from many different countries. The changed context has created an enabling environment for the emergence of medical tourism as an international business opportunity in many developing countries.

Medical tourism is likely to be affected by a host of factors including globalization-led institutional, technological and socioeconomic changes. It operates within the institutional framework of the national health system and maintains a relationship with the public health facilities and hospitals. In theory, global competition among the provider hospitals should promote efficiency and quality of care, build new hospitals, attract foreign investments along with patients, and encourage expansion of both private and public health care sectors.

Modern medical tourism began as a survival strategy of some Southeast Asian hospitals after the Asian recession in 1997. Today, it has become a billion dollar global business spanning virtually all continents. In the era of globalization, health care has joined other commodities in having some of its 'production' outsourced to countries with a competitive cost advantage. Medical tourism exemplifies this business approach. Poorer nations export health care expertise and services to patients of wealthier countries when similar services are generally more expensive. In 2007, approximately 750,000 American patients outsourced their medical treatment as part of reducing their cost of care, primarily to health facilities in less developed countries.

The number of patients outsourcing their medical care is expected to continue to increase in coming years. Patients in rich countries will increasingly have choices and options in selecting countries and medical facilities for their treatment. This has promoted competitions among service providers in host countries to build technologically advanced facilities, using both foreign and domestic capital, and to provide internationally accepted quality of service at affordable prices. In many instances, hospitals in host countries had to hire technicians and nurses meeting international qualification standards to remain competitive when such personnel were not available locally. The medical tourism industry is now attempting to target small businesses and health insurance companies in developed countries, in addition to individual clients, to increase customer volume. This strategy seems to be working; it has generated interest among large corporate sectors and legislatures of developed countries as a means of reducing the cost of health care.

For a long time medical tourism was generally considered to be the travel of wealthy patients from a less developed country to the health facilities in more developed and medically advanced countries to get better treatment. But the global market place for health care has changed. Today, medical tourism goes in both directions, from rich and poor countries alike; and has seen developing countries become the primary destinations where high quality affordable healthcare is available. According to a 2008 estimate, the medical tourism business is in operation in 28 countries globally. Currently, the most popular destinations for medical tourism are countries once characterized as "third world" such as Thailand, India, Malaysia, Singapore, the Philippines, Jordan, Turkey, Hungary, Mexico, Cuba, Chile and South Africa, while a few other medical tourist hubs are emerging in Dubai and Eastern Europe. Table 1 shows the size of the medical tourism trade in terms of patients treated, earnings generated and the type of services provided by hospitals in major host countries.

Table 1. Medical Tourism: Estimated Patients Treated and Money Spent in selected Countries

Country	Patients treated	Estimated earnings (US$)	Major services provided
Thailand	900,000 (in 2008)	850 million (2008)	Cosmetic surgery, organ transplants, dental treatment, joint replacements
India	450,000 (in 2007)	480 million (2005)	Cardiac surgery, joint replacements, eye surgery
Malaysia	350,000 (in 2007)	43 million (2005)	Cardiology, cardiothoracic surgery, cosmetic surgery
Singapore	410,000 (in 2006)	560 million (2004)	Liver transplants, joint replacements, cardiac surgery

Thailand has pioneered medical tourism in its modern form and is still leading in terms of number of patients treated and foreign exchange earnings. The country has the advantage of having a large tourist industry and infrastructure already in place to attract tourists from across the globe. One feature of Thai medical tourism is its flexibility in pricing for services to accommodate the means of its customers. Also, Thai international hospitals have adopted a corporate philosophy to promote customer satisfaction. The costs of medical services are often packaged with stays at oceanfront resorts, guided tours and nightclub cabarets in Bangkok to attract international patients.

India entered the medical tourism market late but is quickly catching up with other leading countries to become a leading global health care provider. According to one report, Indian hospitals treated approximately 450,000 international patients in 2007 and earned about USD 480 million in 2005. The main strength of the Indian approach is its capacity to provide medical services at the lowest cost among all international health care providers. India has other advantages including a large pool of physicians, many of whom were trained in the UK or USA, English is widely spoken in the country and several hospitals are accredited by the Joint Commission International (JCI). The most popular services of the Indian medical tourism industry are heart surgeries, joint replacements, hip resurfacing, cataract operations, cosmetic surgery, dentistry and gallstone removal. Like Thailand, India has always been a tourist destination that also offered alternative medical treatments like Ayurveda, Yoga and Kairali.

Malaysia also began its active role in the medical tourism industry after the financial crisis of 1997 caused a drop in the number of domestic patients visiting private hospitals. These hospitals were forced to search for alternative patients overseas, through government trade missions and other promotional activities. While starting late compared to its regional competitors, Malaysia quickly moved to expand its business and generated about USD 43 million in 2005. It is expected to generate at least USD 55 million in 2010 (ESCAP). Popular treatments that the country offers include cardiac and cardiothoracic surgeries, radiotherapy and radiology. Most of the international patients it received in 2006 were from Indonesia (72%), Singapore (10%), Japan (5%) and West Asia (2%) (ESCAP 2009). The Ministry of Health has actively coordinated with about 34 private international hospitals, tour agencies and other relevant bodies to promote medical travel in Malaysia.

Although costs of medical care are higher than in Thailand or India, Singapore has a reputation for high-quality medical facilities and is well known for delivering cutting-edge medical treatment, including surgeries such as liver and heart transplants and complex neurosurgical procedures. It attracted more than 410,000 international patients from 60 countries to generate more than USD 560 million in 2006. Singapore is home to three high quality hospitals accredited by the JCI.

Several other developing countries such as the Philippines, Jordan, South Africa and Mexico have been either quick to recognize the opportunities of medical travel or are expanding its already developed infrastructure to get their share of the fast expanding global health care market. Given their high-quality medical professionals and competitive cost of service, they are working toward becoming the next medical care destinations in their regions. Since the early 1990s, Jordan has been trying to become the medical hub for the Arab world, to treat patients primarily from the Middle East. The government provides incentives for private investment in the health sector. Its hospitals have specialized in cardiac surgery, spinal injuries, cornea transplants and alternative medicine. Several health facilities in Jordan are formally linked with prestigious hospitals in Europe and North America as a strategy to become more attractive to international patients.

Among the Latin American countries, Cuba attempted to become a world medical power in the 1980s. The Cuban government created a company to arrange medical treatments and travel for foreign patients and hosted thousands of patients each year from Latin America, the Caribbean, Russia, and the United Kingdom. The Cuban hospitals have gained a reputation in ophthalmology, joint surgeries, neurology, and treating skin diseases. However, the country could not attract a large number of US patients for geopolitical reasons. Cuba is also somewhat unique amongst countries engaged in medical tourism, as there are no private facilities involved. The Cuban health system from training, to export of health workers, to import of health patients is under public management.

Medical tourism is also being introduced as a business model in countries not very well known for tourism such as South Korea, the UAE, Turkey, Hungary and Costa Rica. A number of Eastern European countries have started providing dental care and plastic surgery for international patients. Chile, as a regional medical hub in Latin America, has attracted patients from Bolivia, Peru, and Ecuador. Several Chilean clinics have established agreements with health care centres and private insurers in other countries in the region as a strategy to promote medical tourism. Mexico has long been popular among US patients seeking dental care and cosmetic surgeries. Turkey has also become a medical tourist destination by providing low cost services and accrediting some of its hospitals with JCI. Several other countries are also trying to attract foreign patients including Argentina, China, Colombia, the Dominican Republic and South Africa. The medical tourism business has adopted multiple export strategies, and comprises a diverse set of countries across the globe. It is gradually expanding to provide services in all medical procedures.

Driving Forces of Medical Tourism

Medical tourism providers adopted an approach that most multinational and corporate business enterprises follow in terms of designing marketing strategies, pricing, branding, management and maintaining the quality of services. This approach, along with increasing global integration of businesses, and the cost and wait-time crises in western health care systems, created opportunities for many health facilities in developing countries. Key driving forces pf the growth of medical tourism are discussed below.

Cost-effective Services

The major driving force of medical tourism industry is the provision of cost effective private medical care combined with the attraction of visiting exotic sites in the destination countries. The health care package includes traditional therapies as well as surgical and specialized treatments. The industry is now facilitated by the corporate sector specialized in both medical care and tourism. The industry has a network of professional medical brokerages who reach out to clients with inadequate or no health insurance coverage, seeking inexpensive healthcare from abroad.

The differences in the cost of care for various treatment options between rich and developing countries are substantial. Table 2 indicates that the cost of care in host countries is, on average, only 10% of the cost in rich countries. For example, the cost of open-heart surgery is $70,000 in Britain and up to $150,000 in the US while it's between $3,000 and $10,000 in India's best hospitals. Surgery on both knees costs $7,700 in India while it costs more than twice as much in Britain ($16,950).

Table 2. Comparative Costs of Selected Medical Services (US$)

Procedure	United States	India	Thailand	Singapore
Heart valve replacement	159,000	9,500	10,500	13,000
Heart bypass	122,000	10,000	12,000	20,000
Knee replacement	41,000	8,500	10,000	12,000
Spinal fusion	63,000	5,500	7,000	9,000
Hysterectomy	20,000	3,000	4,500	6,000

Similarly, dental, eye and cosmetic surgeries in rich countries cost three to four times as much as in India or Thailand. The primary reason for such cost differences between the two types of countries has been low wage rates in host countries compared to most of the developed nations. In the face of continuing health care cost increases in developed countries, it is likely that patients, insurers and employers, particularly in countries where employers share the costs of private health insurance, will continue seeking low cost treatment abroad.

The medical tourism industry is modelled to provide cost effective services using relatively low cost health professionals from the provider countries. There are other ways in which service costs are kept low. In most provider countries, malpractice litigation costs are much lower than in most highly developed countries, which has helped to reduce the cost of care. For example, a physician in Thailand pays about $5,000 per year for a liability insurance policy while an American physician needs to pay more than $100,000 annually for the same. The professional liability insurance premium for a surgeon in India is only 4% of what it is in the US.

Hospitals in developed countries have to follow detailed health care regulations while health care regulations in most provider countries are quite flexible and business-friendly. In the provider countries, hospitals can employ physicians directly to provide a certain number of hours per month in return for a guaranteed fixed fee a practice prohibited in many Western countries. The provider hospitals can also hire reputed and popular physicians as part-time consultants to attract more customers from abroad.

The proliferation of advanced medical technologies and increasing public demands for long-term health care has increased the cost of care in most developed countries, regardless of the market-based (the U.S.), social insurance (Canada, France, Germany, Japan), national health service (Finland, New Zealand, Norway, Sweden, U.K.), or hybrid (Italy, Spain) models of health care financing and provision. Unlike the developing world, patients in the developed world spend only a fraction in out of pocket payments on health care, with the remaining paid by insurers, employers and government. As a result, providers face less competition to keep prices low.

Insurance Coverage

Lack of partial coverage of health insurance in most developed countries is another important driving force in deciding to choose a foreign country for medical care. The number of people without health insurance coverage in the US was estimated as 45 million in 2003. In addition, lack of insurance for dental care and delay for some medical interventions such as orthopaedic operations, spinal surgery ophthalmologic, knee and hip replacements are a serious problem in Canada and many countries in Western Europe. The growing uninsured or underinsured patients in rich industrialized countries along with the rapid increase of healthcare costs has stimulated patients to travel overseas for affordable healthcare. The recent economic recession has led to an increase in the number of uninsured persons in the US and left a large population needing affordable healthcare with little choice but to go abroad for major treatments.

Choices

The medical tourism model promotes patient choice by providing access to a set of service packages with variant costs and quality not found in developed countries. It also expedites access to care, when needed, by substantially reducing waiting periods in some countries for services from public facilities. The model provides opportunities for such surgical procedures as face-lifts, hair transplants, dental treatment and liposuction, as well as nonsurgical procedures such as hair removal most of which are not covered by health insurance and are either expensive or severely restricted for legal reasons in most developed countries. Other choices include opportunities to select destinations (countries), providers (hospitals and physicians) and the types of services based on their expertise and costs of care.

Waiting Time

A large number of international medical travellers have been from such developed countries as Canada and the United Kingdom where health care is under the public domain. The primary reason for those patients to travel abroad is to avoid long waiting times for non-elective surgery and other critical procedures in their own countries. According to an estimate, nearly 900,000 Britons are waiting at any given time for admission to National Health Service hospitals where shortages of capacities force the cancellation of more than 50,000 operations each year. Despite the small improvement in 2007, the total wait time remains high in Canada, both historically and internationally. On average, Canadians are still waiting 121 days or more on average for necessary medical treatment and the wait time is still increasing.

One study reports that the cumulative economic cost of waiting in excess of recommended wait times for joint replacement surgery, cataract surgery, coronary artery bypass graft and MRI scans to be $14.8 billion in Canada even if additional $4.4 billion loss of revenues as a result of reduced economic activity is not counted. In addition, the long wait contributes to unrecognized costs such as physical impairment and anxiety, and physical and psychological pain and suffering that cannot be measured. Wealthy Canadian patients found medical travel as an alternative for surgical procedures in such countries as India, Thailand, Malaysia or the Philippines where they can get the services almost immediately.

Access to Technology

Increased access to information flow regarding medical travel and the pleasure of travel overseas has also significantly contributed to the growth of medical tourism. Most of the international health providers as well as their brokerages have their own websites that facilitate a variety of services. Patients can learn about options, compare costs, select hospitals, make travel arrangements and can contact providers and medical specialists for informed choices. Websites also provide such information as hospital accreditation, doctor's credentials, patient testimonials in addition to cost of treatment and logistics. International hospitals in developing countries use electronic medical records to store and access patient files before discussing the procedures with potential patients via conference call. Medical tourism providers use a business model that combines the personalized services of the hotel industry where tasks and procedures have been streamlined for the highest efficiency.

Innovative Services

Provision of quality assured, often atypical, specialized medical care in international hospitals is another important determinant of the growing popularity of medical travel abroad. Medical care providers in Thailand, for example, have a reputation for cosmetic surgery and dental procedures. Indian hospitals are well known for hip resurfacing technology a procedure that requires a shorter rehabilitation period compared to total hip replacement as suggested in most Western hospitals. Some Indian hospitals offer advanced treatments that are not yet approved in the West such as robot assisted joint replacement. For renal care and kidney transplants with affordable prices, the choice for many patients is the Philippines. Providers in Singapore, where the cost of medical services is relatively higher than neighbouring medical tourist hubs, emphasize complex cases (such as separation of conjoined twins) or the highest quality care to attract medical tourists from developed nations, and wealthy patients from less developed Asian countries who used to travel to reputable medical institutions in Europe or North America. The medical tourism industry offers a relaxing vacation period following the medical procedure in their package. For many western medical tourists, a trip to Thailand or India with some travel and adventure carries extra benefits of getting pleasure.

One positive and significant aspect of the medical tourism model is the opportunity of provider countries to expand their health infrastructure and health human resource base. Wider political issues have also redirected medical travellers to other destinations to seek out health care. The US was a preferred destination for many affluent patients from the Middle East prior to the attack on the World Trade Centre on 11 September 2001. The subsequent tightening of entry requirements in the US (and in many other Western countries) has diverted a large share of the medical tourism business to other destinations. This has created an opportunity for health facilities in

Jordan to position themselves to receive much of the diverted patient load and assume a role as regional referral centre for patients from neighbouring countries. On the other hand, Cuba, although entering the market in the 1980s, with the potential to lead the business, did not flourish as expected because of its political isolation in the region and travel restrictions imposed by some countries.

Quality of Care

Given that accreditation is a vital issue in choosing a hospital for health care by many patients in the West, most of the provider hospitals in the developing countries are now accredited either by the Joint Commission International (JCI) or the International Standards Organization (ISO). Some provider countries have adopted their own accreditation standards to reassure potential patients about their high quality health care. A few of them were affiliated with prestigious Western universities or health care systems to become more attractive to international patients. In many cases, the physicians are trained and certified in the West, to ensure the safety of the potential patients as well as to attract more international patients to their facilities. Intense competition among the international health providers to demonstrate the quality and expertise of their professional staff can have a lasting positive effect on the growth in medical tourism.

Provision of Ethical and Legal Medical Services

The main driving force behind the promotion of medical tourism is to maximize profits by providing health services that can be bought off the shelf from the lowest priced provider anywhere in the globe. The approach, therefore, is not likely to encourage the health care market forces to follow internationally accepted standards, governmental regulations, patients' rights, or legal and ethical issues. It would be difficult, if not impossible, to develop and implement internationally recognized agreements regarding oversight, care provision, ethics and legal recourse. One important feature of the medical tourism market is the provision of services that are either illegal in many developed countries, not paid for by insurance companies (such as face-lifts, hair transplants, dental treatment and liposuction) or which have to go through long legal procedures to get those services (such as surrogacy and organ transplant).

Reproductive (surrogacy) tourism provides a woman with a chance to experience motherhood if she is unable to become pregnant and give birth by natural means. The process is not only costly but is also ridden with many legal hurdles in most developed countries. These factors push many couples to explore alternative countries and facilities providing surrogate mothers. Although this service can be bought in many countries, India has become most successful in providing reproductive outsourcing because surrogacy is legal in India, where a surrogate mother can easily sign away rights to the child without facing any legal problems. Also, it takes much less time to take delivery of the child, compared to 2-4 years in UK. The cost of surrogacy process ranges between \$20,000 to \$35,000 in India, which includes doctor fees, medicines, prenatal care, delivery, legal charges as well as surrogate compensation; the process may cost between \$30,000 to \$100,000 in those developed countries where it is allowed.

Improvements in medical technology have resulted in an unprecedented interest in body contouring as a form of aesthetic surgery, such as abdominoplasty, rhinoplasty or bariatric surgery. The pregnancy-stretched abdomen can now be brought back to an almost pre-pregnancy state, nose shape can be improved and obesity (where diet plans and work-outs fail) can be reduced through surgical procedures. Most of these cosmetic surgeries are not covered by medical insurance in the West and are very expensive. Thailand, India and Mexico have become the cosmetic tourism hubs. Customers have come primarily from the US, Canada, Britain and other European nations. One source estimates that about 29,000 British went overseas for cosmetic surgery and spent USD 156 million in 2007.

Thesevere shortage of human organs for transplant has led to an international organ trade. Although some countries, such as India, have made the sale of human organs a criminal offense (the 1994 Indian Human Organs Transplantation Act), nearly 10 per cent of all transplantations in the world (about 93,000 kidney, liver and heart transplants each year) are estimated to have been carried out illegally. The Istanbul Declaration in 2008 called a halt to these unethical activities and urged safe and accountable practices to protect poor people from the exploitation inherent in organ sales, however, critics suggest that expansion of medical tourism will further promote an organ-selling spree among desperately poor countries. India, Pakistan,

China, the Philippines, Iraq, Egypt, Turkey, Brazil, Bolivia, Peru and East European countries are commonly cited organ-exporting countries, where organs from local donors are regularly transplanted in foreigners through sale and purchase. On the other hand, Australia, Canada, Israel, Japan, Oman, Saudi Arabia and the USA are reported as major organ-importing countries.

Organ suppliers are generally very poor, mostly women and vulnerable people living in the poverty-stricken regions of the world who can either be easily motivated or coerced. A study reports that 71 per cent of such providers lived below the poverty line, 71 per cent were female and 96 per cent had to sell their organs to pay off their household debt. Most of the organ suppliers experienced deterioration of health after donation and became unable to do labour intensive jobs. Medical transplant is thus considered by some as a "globalized apartheid medicine" since it benefits the rich patients generally from the developed countries over the poor and vulnerable who have no choice.

Medical Tourism: Disparities and Opportunities

In an increasingly globalized world where financially capable patients have wider choices and opportunities to go abroad for health services, the growth of medical tourism appears to be inevitable. Privatization of health care, diffusion in information technology, fewer restrictions on movement and low cost air travel have expanded the scope of travelling abroad for health care. While previously only the rich and the famous could afford to be medical tourists, medical tourism is now accessible to a larger section of the population particularly in the developed countries. Not much is known about the implications of medical tourism as very few rigorous studies have examined this issue. While medical tourism has been a boon for some people in destination countries and for those medical tourists able to afford such services, from a public health perspective it is mixed blessing.

Development of Health Infrastructure

Medical tourism has the potential to create opportunities to boost gross domestic product and to create a more favourable balance of trade by lowering the fiscal deficit of the national economy. As a major source of foreign exchange, it can stimulate overall economic growth including tourism, transport, pharmaceuticals, hotels, food suppliers to hospitals and restaurants, and create more jobs in the tourism industry. It improves the image and reputation of the country, helps create international bonds with citizens of other nations, and acts as a role model of an efficient provider for the public health sector.

Such arguments, however, are contested or challenged in several points. Evidence suggests that economic development programs rarely create opportunities for the poor and disadvantaged. Introduction of high tech., medical facilities may, in fact, simply reduce the employment opportunities for the labour-intensive job market. The creation and expansion of large and hightech., health facilities may wrongly be perceived as 'development of the health sector' in the public's eyes to draw their attention away from faltering public health systems.

Expansion of medical tourism emphasizes building only large specialized hospitals to enhance their capacity and income beyond the limited domestic 'market' or what is needed for most of the populations. It has been argued that increasing emphasis on technology driven tertiary care for foreigners may potentially have distorted the healthcare landscape in these countries and, thereby, have deprived their own native-born poor populations.

The medical tourism sector has been reported to be subsidized by the government while public health expenditure has consistently been reduced in some provider countries. In several countries, the private hospitals built for the medical tourists receive special tax benefits in return for their commitment to provide a certain amount of free medical services for the poor patients of the localities. Such agreements have never materialized. However, others argue that the private sector cannot and should not be blamed for the lack of access to health care for the poor and disadvantaged populations as the poor were neglected by their public health systems long before the medical tourism model developed.

Equity in Health Care Access

Medical tourism has been criticized for the creation of a two-tier system of healthcare delivery by broadening the gap between haves and have-nots, and building impressive hightech hospitals that serve only the needs of affluent outsiders. It has also been argued that medical tourism could potentially divide health care systems by diverting larger public sector funds to implement policies that are biased in favour of their business, thereby aggravating inequalities in health care access. As Woodward et al. points out "it (medical tourism) may also divert human resources from public services to more profitable services for the elite or foreign markets, thus reducing staffing levels, lowering staff quality, and/or raising salary costs for the public sector." The poor may have less access to healthcare because it is either too expensive for them or not available where they live. It should be noted, however, that although cheaper by most Western standards, the costs of private hospitals that treat medical tourists have always been out of reach for the majority of the poor within destination countries. This raises the question to the argument that medical tourism may lead to increasing health disparities.

It can be argued that access to care by the poor will be affected by medical tourism for the short-term only if appropriate measures are taken to create a space for the poor to access the high quality health care that medical tourism could provide close to their home. There are many ways to create opportunities for the poor. One widely known option has been the provision of cross-subsidies for poor patients by the rich. However, generating revenues through the cross-subsidisation process has been difficult to implement. Evidence suggests that Indian private hospitals, which provide services to international patients, have failed to fulfil their expected role to treat local poor for free in return for government subsidies. On the other hand, Cuba's Servimed is an example where it is claimed that many of the profits from foreign patients get reinvested in local health care provision. Another promising option is the creation of a social business oriented health care industry where a substantial amount of the profits goes to benefit the poor and underserved.

The argument that private hospitals serving medical tourists will continue to treat only foreign patients is improbable, since the revenue generated from foreign patients will remain well below the running cost of most of these hospitals. Such hospitals have focused on the affluent and financially well-off population of their own countries as a strategy to expand their customer base. Availability of the advanced medical care in those hospitals with relatively lower cost has, in fact, expanded access to high quality medical care for the population able to afford such care.

Medical tourism has the potential to accelerate health technology transfer to less developed countries. With the expansion of medical tourism, some of the large hospitals in the host countries have transformed themselves to become centres of excellence and regional hubs for advanced medical care. The newly gained status and strength of these hospitals have the potential not only to reduce the dominance of major Western medical facilities but also to contribute to a reduction in global inequality by providing high quality care for clients in the regions. In the developed world with a large proportion of the population without health insurance, the growth in medical tourism might contribute to a reduction in health disparities in those countries by creating opportunities for such persons to receive essential medical care abroad.

Mobility of Health Professionals

The effects of the expansion of medical tourism on the mobility of medical professionals are unclear. It may be argued that the classic model of brain-drain, where medical professionals from poorer developing countries move to wealthier developed nations for more opportunities to work, higher pay and professional development, will be affected by the growth of the modern form of medical tourism. Fewer health professionals will have reason to seek greater practice opportunities abroad, although other dynamics are also at play.

Hospitals catering to foreign patients will continue searching for highly skilled professionals to raise the quality of care and reputation of the facilities to attract new customers. This recruitment drive is likely to accelerate:

- internal migration of medical professionals primarily from the public facilities to hospitals for foreign patients,
- reverse brain-drain of professionals from the developed countries to their home country hospitals, and
- migration of professionals from the neighbouring countries to newly built medical tourism hub centres in the region.

As expected, internal brain-drain has been reported in Thailand, creating a shortage of doctors in the public hospitals in Bangkok because of the higher pay offered at Bumrungrad, a major hospital in the region that treats medical tourists. This has prompted criticism of medical tourism on the speculation that the flooding of foreigners into developing countries would divert money and expertise from the public health facilities in the rural areas to further worsen the care for disadvantaged people. At the same time this is seen as a distraction from the need to cut costs and improve quality in rich-world health systems. Nonetheless, the external brain drain has been somewhat replaced by an internal brain drain where more doctors have left public health facilities to work in private large hospitals. Although it is difficult to get a clear picture of the flows of internal brain-drain of health workers due to a lack of monitoring and formal reporting systems, it has been observed that medical tourism has encouraged such movements. The argument of the negative effect of internal brain-drain, however, has been countered by the contention that the growth of medical tourism may have reduced the flow of health care professionals from provider countries to the developed world.

Brain-drain of health professionals from the developing to developed countries is well documented. It is claimed that medical tourism, in being capable of providing attractive salaries to its skilled professionals, has the capacity to reverse the flow. Although debatable, anecdotal evidence suggests that a large pool of highly skilled medical professionals trained in developed countries were attracted to return to their home countries, as they found it lucrative and more satisfying to work at home. In addition, returning professionals had gained experience of working in major medical facilities in developed countries with international goodwill. Critics, however, argue that such reverse brain-drain would not help patients of their home countries because they would use infrastructure and other resources of their own country to serve the foreigners thus depriving their own people.

A large influx of international health travellers to provider countries would likely raise the demand for more private hospitals or expansion of the existing health infrastructure. This will require more health professionals and the potential loss of more doctors not only from the public sector, but also from the least developed neighbouring countries. In other words, expansion of medical tourism may have negative effects on poor patients in public facilities in the region who are in need of care and support.

Quality and Safety

Intense competition among health facilities in the global health market is likely to promote technological advances and improve medical infrastructure in their own institutions. Medical tourism encourages hospitals to invest in high-quality facilities, cutting-edge technology and human resources to attract international patients. It has been reported that the best hospitals in Asia and Latin America now rival or surpass many hospitals in the rich world for safety and quality. The facilities can provide better care for the affluent local population and promote equity in access to private care for patients who otherwise would not have access to such facilities and services. Upgraded facilities can have a demonstration effect on the national health system by raising the overall standard of health care and forcing public health facilities to invest more to improve their quality of care.

Issues of Waste Management

The problem of medical waste management in the provider countries, as a result of a large influx of surgical patients from overseas, has already become a serious concern, but remains largely unnoticed in the medical literature. The local people are not generally aware of the threats they are exposed to living close to medical waste dumps. One study reports that a bed in a hospital generates on average 1 kg waste per day, out of which 10-15 per cent is infectious, 5 per cent hazardous and the rest general. Given that most developing countries have no proper medical waste management system, the problem of medical waste management is likely to grow with the promotion of medical tourism.

Governance of Medical Tourism

One of the greatest achievements of modern times is the increasing longevity of human life. With population aging, the demand for medical and long-term care has gradually been increasing, particularly in developed countries. Globalization of health care systems has created risks and challenges even while opening new opportunities for the provision of better and more affordable medical care for a larger population. With the rising costs of production, health services in many developed countries are now increasingly outsourced. Relatively poor or uninsured patients of the rich countries are now moving abroad, mostly to developing countries, to receive health care within reasonable costs, although often by ignoring the risk of quality of services they receive. This trend is likely to increase over time as medical tourism becomes an accepted part of the solution to high health care costs or long wait times to receive care in the West. Medical tourism will expand further once governments allow health insurers and employers to extend their coverage abroad, although this expansion may generate additional health disparities in the provider countries.

Expansion of medical tourism appears to be inevitable within the context of a new global economic order. What is needed is to create a medical tourism governance structure by the key stakeholders in this sector such as representative of the governments, medical care providers, employer groups, pharmaceutical companies, health insurers, international medical brokers, and the patients. They will carefully consider all relevant issues such as the experience and achievements of medical tourism approach so far, expectations from expanded medical tourism, and identification of the existing problems and potential obstacles to reaching targets, impact on the health systems of provider countries, and equity of health care for those worse off in developing countries. Given the lack of evidence of the outcome of expanded medical tourism in recent decades, it would be difficult at this juncture to set out policy options for the future of medical tourism.

Auditing

Managing risks that medical tourism may create while preserving benefits it can offer requires a clear understanding of how it affects the cost of health care and the quality of services. Also, it is important to monitor the long-term effects of medical tourism on access to and utilization of services, efficiency and effectiveness of care, and health equity in developing countries, and ensure that monitoring results are fed effectively into decision-making processes at the national and international levels.

Conducting a global audit to understand the current status of medical tourism and developing a routine monitoring system to keep track of its growth and effects would provide an evidence base on which informed decisions could be made. Several relevant issues remain to be understood before developing a good governance system of medical tourism. Some of these are existing mechanisms to monitor the quality of care at medical tourism facilities, current practices and responsibilities of managing legal and malpractice issues, maintaining privacy of patients, continuity of care or patient follow-up after returning to home countries, and effects of medical tourism on the access to health services in both provider and recipient countries. Also, an appraisal to look at the current structure, process and outcome of the medical tourism business would help in devising a future strategy for its growth. At present, no legitimate authority, recognized by the stakeholders, exists that could develop quality and safety standards for medical tourism, a global database to monitor trends, and a set of criteria for auditing or reviewing the medical tourism business on a regular basis.

Regulations

In the absence of regulatory systems and guarantees of rights or protections, patients are taking a calculated risk by seeking medical care abroad. One of the inherent weaknesses of the medical tourism trade is that no single authority has jurisdiction over the patients, health providers, referral networks, employers and insurers.

With the expansion of business at the global level, the system calls for a set of policies under a regulatory framework and establishment of a legitimate authority to develop, modify and implement those policies. The development of both structure and scope of the proposed regulatory framework requires a systematic review of the medical tourism sector and intensive discussion with the stakeholders.

The scope of the proposed agency or authority would be to protect public interest by creating and monitoring guidelines for international health trade, advocating standardization for the qualification of physicians and other medical professionals, granting licenses and accreditation for international hospitals, regulating the activities of international health brokers, employers and insurers, and assisting in sharing information, outcomes reporting and other aspects of the medical tourism trade among stakeholders.

Several national and international healthcare groups have understood the need of having such an authority and are working to develop an effective system to respond to the fast transforming healthcare practice, technologies and medical delivery procedures in the world. The program of International Health Regulations (IHR) of WHO is already in place to respond to acute public health risks that have the potential to cross borders and threaten people worldwide. The WHO, as a legitimate and widely accepted international agency, may take the responsibility of functioning as a provider of knowledge and evidence, and initiate the development of policy guidelines for medical tourism governance.

Reducing the Disparities

Making medical tourism work to reduce health inequity in both rich and poor countries requires fundamental changes in the current form of medical tourism. A clear understanding of needed changes calls for systematic studies on the impact of the expansion of medical tourism on the diffusion of advanced medical technologies in the developing world and their effects on access to care for poor and disadvantaged patients living in provider countries.

Extending the benefits of improved health services geographically means that both private and public hospitals in provider countries coordinate in ways that maximize the opportunities medical tourism has created. This may mean substantial changes in institutional arrangements such as the removal of legal obstacles for the expansion of the private sector, provision of insurance coverage for international patients and formulation of policies regarding patient safety and malpractices. Promotion of such collaboration among various stakeholders is likely to enhance the financial capacity of the public health sector, help improve the standard of services of public facilities and improve availability and quality of services for the public at large. However, it remains to be clearly understood how, to what extent and under what mechanism those stakeholders with opposing interests would work together to reach a common goal.

Provider hospitals should maintain a diversified and balanced portfolio of local and international patients in order to avoid the excessive reliance on revenue from international patients and business risks. One study suggests that the provision of providing services to local clients would minimize, to some degree, the risks associated with dependency on international patients. Like normal tourism business, international health providers should be encouraged to promote effective, but low cost medical facilities for average patients. This would likely provide wider choices and better opportunities not only for patients from abroad but for the local population as well.

Both private and public health insurance carriers in developed countries should be encouraged to extend their coverage of services overseas. They should be provided incentives to encourage beneficiaries to use offshore facilities for expensive surgical procedures and take advantage of low-cost treatments.

References

Arellano ABR. (2007). Patients Without Borders: The Emergence of Medical Tourism. *International Journal of Health Services* 37(1):193–198.

Bookman MZ, Bookman KR. (2007). *Medical Tourism in Developing Countries*. New York: Palgrave Macmillan.

Connell J. (2006). Medical tourism: Sea, sun, sand and … surgery. *Tourism Management* 27:1093–1100.

Deloitte. (2008). *Medical Tourism. Consumers in Search of Value*. Washington DC: Deloitte Centre for Health Solutions.

ESCAP. (2009). *Medical Travel in Asia and the Pacific. Challenges and Opportunities*. Bangkok: United Nations Economic and Social Commission for Asia and the Pacific.

Herrick DM. 2007. Medical Tourism: Global Competition in Health Care. *NCPA Policy Report No. 304*, November 2007.

Smith K. (2008). Medical Tourism: For Richer or Poorer. *Paper presented at Ownership & Appropriation, a joint conference of the ASA, the ASAANZ and the AAS*, 8th - 12th December 2008, University of Auckland, New Zealand.

WHO (2000). *The World Health Report 2000 – Health Systems: Improving Performance*. Geneva: WHO.

4

Risks and Opportunities of Medical Tourism

"Medical tourism" is not entirely new. Bartha Knoppers and Sonia LeBris coined the term "procreative tourism" in 1991 to describe the practice of patients exercising "their personal reproductive choices in other less restrictive states." Moreover, foreign citizens have sought medical care in the United States and other countries with advanced medicine for decades. For example, California has been a popular worldwide destination for reproductive tourists because it offers advanced technology, medical expertise, and relatively permissive fertility laws.

Medical tourism has exploded in recent years, aided by globalization in the health services industry. But globalization has only recently permeated health care. Traditionally, geographic, economic, and cultural barriers have made health care stubbornly local. Gradually, countries have opened their borders. Now there are thriving international markets for health care professionals, telemedicine, medical technology, and drugs. More recently, the U.S. health care industry has started outsourcing a number of related tasks, including insurance claim processing, medical reporting, clinical trials, and diagnostic test interpretations. The latest and perhaps most important segment to succumb to globalization is the market for patients. In 2003, an estimated 350,000 patients from various countries travelled to Cuba, India, Jordan, Malaysia, Singapore, and Thailand for medical care. In 2005, over 55,000 Americans visited Bumrungrad Hospital in Bangkok for medical care. In India alone, the number of medical tourists visiting the country tripled between 2002 and 2005, and is expected to rise by 600% over the next few years.

Reasons of Travelling for Medical Care

Patients generally seek medical care abroad for one of two reasons: either they do not have access to a particular treatment, or they cannot afford it, in their own country.

Issues of Access

Historically, patients have travelled overseas when a particular medical treatment is not available where they live. First, local laws may prohibit a medical procedure as immoral or unethical, which occurs most often with reproductive medicine. For example, patients in Europe flock to Belgium and Italy for in vitro fertilization (IVF) treatments because these two countries "have no or very little legislation concerning medically assisted reproduction." Many patients visit from France, Germany, or the Netherlands, whose governments impose various restrictions on IVF treatments. Every year, 7,000 women from Ireland travel to England for abortions because abortion is illegal in Ireland.

Second, certain treatments may not be available when they have not been approved by regulators. In the United States, the Food and Drug Administration (FDA) must approve most medical technologies before they can be marketed. Many believe that a strict, lengthy FDA approval process delays the availability of cutting-edge medical technologies that are widely used overseas. American patients obtained a hip resurfacing surgery in Europe, Asia, and India that FDA had not approved until recently. Patients are keenly aware that foreign regulators have approved certain procedures that FDA has not. A patient that travelled to India for heart surgery testified to the U.S. Senate that "[p]rocedures are often available in developing countries years before the FDA approves them in the U.S." Whether it is wise or not, patients travel overseas for procedures that have not been approved by their domestic regulators.

Third, even in the absence of restrictive laws or regulations, non-governmental actors may ban certain medical procedures not as a matter of law, but as a matter of fact. Physicians, hospitals, and particularly insurers can decide to make a procedure unavailable. For example, in countries that do not legislate reproductive treatments, "each doctor and clinic decides autonomously whether to provide a certain type of treatment and whether to offer a service to a certain type of patient."

In Mississippi, only one clinic is willing to perform abortions, even though decisions by the U.S. Supreme Court currently prohibit states from banning all abortion procedures outright. Perhaps more common is where a health insurer refuses to cover a particular treatment, whether because the insurer deems the procedure to be immoral, experimental (despite FDA approval), or not worth the expense compared to more established treatments. Thus, an insurer's decision to not cover a particular fertility treatment could lead those with insurance to travel overseas. The absence of laws and regulations leaves a void that non-governmental actors can fill at their discretion. Their decisions may drive patients to forum shop.

Fourth, certain procedures may be unavailable in certain countries that lack the requisite medical technology, expertise, or infrastructure. For example, patients from Bolivia, Peru, and Ecuador travel to Chile for its superior medical care. Indian hospitals attract 50,000 patients each year from Bangladesh. Jordanian hospitals attract medical tourists from Yemen, Sudan, Libya, Algeria, Tunisia, and Iraq. Since the 1970s, the EU recognized that some member states may have medical capabilities that other states lack, and has required states to permit their citizens to travel to other states for medical care when the treatment cannot be given domestically in a medically appropriate timeframe. Thus, variations in medical sophistication between countries can encourage medical tourism.

Finally, foreign doctors provide an outlet to patients in countries with socialized medicine that may have to wait several months for certain medical treatments. In the United Kingdom in 2004, the National Health Service (NHS) expected 41,000 patients to wait at least six months for various surgeries. In response, the NHS began sending patients to France, Spain, and Germany for orthopedic, eye, and other surgeries. As noted above, EU regulations require member states to reimburse for the medical treatments their citizens receive in other states if there is an "undue delay" in the patient's home country, given the patient's medical condition. Based on these regulations, the European Court of Justice recently required the NHS to reimburse a U.K. resident for a hip replacement she obtained in France, even though she failed to obtain prior authorization from the NHS. Thus, patients in countries with socialized medicine may travel to bypass long waiting lists.

Issues of Cost

Although most patients have travelled overseas for procedures that were not available, for one reason or another, where they resided, a new breed of patients is travelling to take advantage of the significant cost discrepancies between countries. In effect, these patients are engaging in international health care arbitrage.

Unsurprisingly, Americans can easily find less expensive medical care overseas. A World Bank study found that the costs of health care and insurance "are significantly higher in the U.S. than in a number of other countries." We spend far more on health care than even our peer countries. In 2000, we spent 44% more per capita on health care than the next highest spending country, Switzerland. That year, we spent 13% of our GDP on health care, significantly higher than Australia (8.3%), Canada (9.1%), Japan (7.8%), and the United Kingdom (7.3%).

These discrepancies are driven in substantial part by the cost of individual medical procedures. For example, the World Bank found that inpatient knee surgery costs over $10,000 on average in the United States, but is only $1,500 at the top hospitals in Hungary and India. A coronary artery bypass graft costs over $35,000 in the United States but is less than $9,000 (including travel expenses) at the top hospitals in India and Thailand. The WHO found that the cost of medical treatment in developing countries such as India can be 3–10% of the cost in the United States.

The World Bank compared the costs of the most common surgical procedures in the United States and in 20 developing countries. The authors used several criteria to identify medical procedures that patients could easily obtain overseas. For example, they searched for low-risk, nonemergency treatments with quick recovery periods. The authors applied these criteria to a list of 230 of the most commonly performed surgeries in U.S. hospitals and compared the mean and median prices for fifteen procedures in twenty countries. Factoring in the cost of round-trip airfare, the World Bank concluded that the United States could save $1.4 billion if only 10% of patients travelled for these fifteen procedures. Half of these savings ($690 million per year) would accrue to the Medicare program.

The United States is enamoured with expensive new drugs, devices, and procedures. It has a steadily aging population, though European populations are older and spend much less on health care. The Americans notorious for their medical malpractice system, but malpractice accounts for less than 2% of our overall health care costs, and awards are markedly higher in Canada and Britain. The most powerful explanation may be labour costs. They pay health care professionals more than any other Organization for Economic Cooperation and Development (OECD) country. According to the primary U.S. agency responsible for health care financing, the Centres for Medicare and Medicaid Services (CMS), nearly 70% of inpatient hospital costs are labour-related. Thus, countries with lower labour costs logically can offer medical care at significantly lower prices.

The US demand for less expensive medical care only increases as more Americans lose insurance coverage. Currently, nearly forty-seven million Americans are uninsured, over eight million of whom are in households that earn $75,000 or more per year. In 2002 and 2003, nearly eighty-two million non-elderly Americans were uninsured at some point, representing one-third of that population. For many patients, treatment overseas is the best option, and for some patients, it is the only option. A medical tourist testified to the U.S. Senate that he paid $6,700 for life-saving heart surgery in India because he could not afford the estimated $200,000 it would have cost in the United States. Similar stories abound. Put simply, a growing number of patients are prepared to travel abroad for medical treatments.

Trends Assisting Medical Tourism

Four broad trends have allowed developing countries to meet the increased demand by foreign patients. First, these countries have dramatically improved the quality of care they can offer, and have become increasingly adept at marketing their services. Second, the Internet allows patients to find foreign providers, and providers can signal their credentials and schedule treatments. Third, the private sector is taking a more active role in health care in many countries, which brings new resources. Finally, several complimentary industries and tasks are being outsourced. These trends suggest that patients will travel more in the coming years.

Improved Quality of Care in Developing Countries

Developing countries are attracting foreign patients because they can offer health care professionals, facilities, and technology that rival the best in the United States. This does not mean that all hospitals in developing countries meet our standards; on average, the quality of health care in the United States is still superior. Rather, the relevant comparison is between the average U.S. hospital and the hospitals in developing countries that attract foreign patients. Here, the quality gap seems to evaporate, insofar as we can measure it. The World Bank found "significant evidence that the upper end of the quality distribution of both professionals and hospitals in several advanced developing countries lies well above the minimum acceptable standards in industrial countries." Developing countries have improved quality in three key areas: medical professionals, facilities, and technology.

First, medical professionals in developing countries increasingly meet Western standards. Many countries are adapting their medical curricula to North American and western European standards, and increasingly offer classes in English. In fact, the United States accepts a large number of foreign students into graduate medical education programs. Over one-quarter of all interns, residents, and fellows in the United States graduated from foreign medical schools. Many of these graduates become board certified in the United States and practice here for years before returning overseas. For example, Bumrungrad Hospital in Bangkok, Thailand, boasts over 200 physicians that were board certified in the United States. Medical professionals are quite mobile most of the global trade in health services is the movement of medical professionals between countries. A quarter of all physicians practicing in the United States in 2004 were educated overseas, and the top eight countries that produce foreign physicians in the United States are all developing countries. Increasingly, patients can leave the United States and still find physicians who are intimately familiar with U.S. medicine.

Second, hospitals in developing countries increasingly meet U.S. standards. Joint Commission International (JCI) has accredited over eighty hospitals and health care facilities in South America, the Caribbean, Asia, India, Africa, and the Middle East. JCI is run by the same organization that accredits U.S. hospitals, the Joint Commission on Accreditation of Healthcare Organizations (JCAHO). Accreditation generally signals that a facility meets minimum standards of competence and quality.

Moreover, JCAHO is governed by major medical trade associations, including the American Medical Association and the American Hospital Association. Hospitals around the world are seeking JCI accreditation, which may help them apply for coverage from U.S. insurers. Thus, patients that leave the United States for medical care increasingly find hospitals that meet U.S. standards.

Many predict that medical tourism will greatly expand as international standards emerge for health care quality, accreditation, and education. For example, several groups have created international standards for health care quality and hospital accreditation. The EU evaluates quality monitoring systems across EU countries. The International Society for Quality in Health Care created a program to align health care standards and accreditation processes internationally. A group of countries even created a program for evaluating the accrediting bodies themselves. Medical education is being standardized by the World Federation for Medical Education and the Institute for International Medical Education, and these standards "are already influencing national and regional systems of recognition and accreditation of medical schools." As various international standards coalesce, developing countries can adopt the same standards as countries with first-rate health systems.

Finally, many developing countries have improved the medical technology they can offer, including procedures and technologies that have yet to be approved by the FDA. Some hospitals in developing countries are even improving biotechnology products made by American and European companies. Foreign hospitals readily advertise these advances. For example, the Wockhardt Hospitals Group in India boasts that it uses the same medical equipment that can be found "in [h]ospitals in New York, London or Sydney." Bumrungrad Hospital in Bangkok advertises that it has two cardiac catheterization laboratories and two cardiac operating theatres. Penang Adventist Hospital in Malaysia is General Electric's Southeast Asia test facility, "one of only a handful of facilities around the globe that receives the next generation of [imaging] equipment before the rest of the medical world." Thus, select hospitals overseas can offer comparably advanced medical technologies.

Communication Technology

The second major trend that facilitates medical tourism is use of the Internet by patients, foreign providers, and intermediaries. The Internet facilitates nearly all facets of medical tourism. Many American patients research medical conditions, providers, products, and treatment options online. Indeed, eighty percent of adult Web users in the United States (136 million people) have used the Internet to search for health information. Searching for health information is the most popular use of the Internet aside from using e-mail and searching for consumer products and services.

Foreign providers have become increasingly savvy and assertive in advertising to foreign patients online. A simple Internet search for "medical tourism" or "surgery abroad" yields hundreds of Web sites for foreign hospitals, clinics, travel agents, medical tourism brokers, and other sites trying to entice foreign patients. Virtually every hospital that caters to foreign patients has an English Web site. And these Web sites are increasingly functional. Many allow patients to schedule treatments, book hotels and airfare, and even contact their surgeons. Patients can also find medical tourism brokers on the Internet that will liaise with foreign hospitals and make travel arrangements.

More importantly, health care providers use the Internet to signal their quality. Virtually every facility with JCI accreditation advertises it on its Web site. Most sites advertise the treatments they offer, their success rates, the technologies they use, the number of physicians they employ that were trained or board certified in Western countries, and the ratio of registered nurses to each foreign patient. Finally, most foreign hospital Web sites either list the prices they charge or provide free quotes on request, bringing unprecedented price transparency to the health services industry. Thus, the Internet not only helps patients and providers connect, but it helps them share key information.

Privatization of Health Care Sectors

The third trend facilitating medical tourism is the increased privatization of foreign health care sectors. Unlike the United States, most countries rely primarily on the government to insure their citizens. But currently, the majority of health services in the world are financed privately. Private insurance is available in virtually all countries, and few governments provide health care services directly anymore. Even in countries with national or socialized health insurance, there is a mix of public and private hospitals.

Currently, an unprecedented number of countries at all levels of development are restructuring their health care systems and reducing their governments roles as health care providers. Public entities are gradually reducing their health spending and selling their health care enterprises. The private sector is filling this void. Governments are inviting more private sector participation in health care and in related sectors such as insurance and telecommunications.

Moreover, governments increasingly see the health care sector as a money-maker, as it generates fresh revenues from abroad. Public hospitals are beginning to reserve a minimum number of private beds for foreign patients. Public officials in Australia claim that the income from treating one foreign patient in a public hospital can be used to treat two or three Australian patients on waiting lists. Private firms have taken notice, and are investing money to increase the number of private beds in public hospitals.

More significantly, privatization is attracting foreign direct investment (FDI). Traditionally, most developing countries limited FDI in the health sector by capping foreign equity investments, imposing discriminatory taxes, enforcing restrictive competition policies, and requiring burdensome economic needs tests and other clearances. Most countries have treated the health industry differently from other industries because they perceive health care to be a public good reserved for the government domain. However, there are new opportunities for FDI as countries privatize their health sectors. Countries have realized that they need FDI to modernize their health care infrastructure. For example, India, Indonesia, Nepal, Maldives, Sri Lanka, and Thailand have opened their health care markets to foreign investors. More foreign investors are establishing hospitals, clinics, diagnostic centres, nursing homes, and treatment centres in developing countries. FDI in hospitals has a considerable impact on local health care infrastructure and helps attract foreign patients. Investors are attracted to FDI in the health sector because of the potentially high rates of return. Thus, as countries privatize health care, they encourage local hospitals and providers to attract lucrative foreign patients.

Globalization of Health Care Services

The fourth major trend that facilitates medical tourism is the globalization of related health care industries. Health care is one of the most rapidly growing markets in the world. Experts expected worldwide health care spending to grow by $800 billion between 2002 and 2005, from $3.2 to $4 trillion. This market includes services and products that make it easier for patients to obtain medical care overseas.

The most obvious example is the global market for health professionals. The medical profession is undeniably global. Over 25% of all physicians, interns, and residents in the United States graduated from foreign medical schools. Foreign-educated nurses comprise a large percentage of nurses practicing in the United States. And other countries' medical professions are similarly diverse. In fact, most of the global trade in health services to date has been the movement of medical professionals between countries. "Doctors without borders" have paved the way for "patients without borders."

The global hospital industry also facilitates medical tourism by creating international hospital chains. Two Singapore-based companies, the Parkway Group and the Raffles Medical Group, have acquired hospitals and established joint ventures with local health care providers in Malaysia, India, Sri Lanka, and the United Kingdom. The

Parkway Group's international hospital chain, Gleneagles International, is now one of the largest health care organizations in Asia. The Raffles Medical Group has agreed to form fifty-fifty joint ventures with Kaiser Permanente throughout Asia. The Apollo Hospitals Group in India has plans to build hospitals in Sri Lanka, Nepal, and Malaysia. And California-based Adventist Health International runs a network of more than 500 Christian not-for-profit hospitals and clinics, led by Penang Adventist Hospital in Malaysia, a major medical tourist destination.

Health care facilities have globalized as countries have privatized and liberalized trade in their health care sectors, and as organizations like the Joint Commission offer international accreditation. Because these hospitals were designed with international standards and patients in mind, their growth has enabled the growth of medical tourism.

The rapid globalization of other industries also facilitates medical tourism, even if the influence is less direct. The global pharmaceutical market has grown between 11– 18% since 2004 in developing countries in Africa, Asia, and Latin America. The WHO predicted the global market for medical devices would grow from $145 billion in 2000 to over $260 billion in 2006. The global market for "telemedicine" and "telehealth" alone is $1.25 trillion and rising. Although health insurance markets in developing countries are quite modest, they should grow as citizens increasingly demand insurance and are able to pay for it. Managed care companies earn billions overseas. U.S. companies have started outsourcing insurance claims processing, which should help cultivate the global health insurance market. Companies from the United States and Europe increasingly outsource their clinical trials. In fact, the global contract research industry, which manages clinical trials for pharmaceutical, medical device, and biotechnology companies, is almost entirely new.

These markets are globalizing health care products, services, and standards. As with the other trends, this trend helps export Western medicine overseas, diminishing the perceived quality gap between domestic and foreign providers, such that the cost differentials become more salient. Patients are learning that they can purchase similar health care products and services overseas at a fraction of the price.

Trends in Global Healthcare Market

As mobile as patients have become, they do not travel to all countries for all procedures. Patients generally receive preventative and emergency care where they live, and some may be too sick or frail to travel. Moreover, not all countries try to attract foreign patients. This section examines the countries that patients visit, the procedures they seek, and the efforts by developing countries to attract foreign patients.

India

India is the fastest growing medical tourist destination. In 2002 and 2003, Indian hospitals treated 150,000 foreign patients, 62,000 of whom travelled to India specifically for medical care. The Confederation of Indian Industry predicts that by 2012, India will generate $2.3 billion per year in revenues from medical tourism. Patients visit India from all over the world, but most often from the Middle East, Europe, and the United States. Patients often visit India for complex procedures, particularly in cardiology, endocrinology, nephrology, neurology, orthopedic surgery, ophthalmology, and urology.

India is positioning itself as a worldwide medical tourist destination. Its government aims to replicate the Thai government's efforts to aggressively market its medical tourism industry. The Ministry of Tourism has called for joint public-private efforts to promote Indian hospitals, and in 2006 formed an interagency task force to promote the industry. The government recently recommended price ranges for common medical treatments in order to keep prices down. Moreover, several states within India have formed public-private medical tourism councils to regulate the industry and market the quality of providers in their regions.

Nevertheless, India faces many of the same problems that other developing countries face. Its legal and regulatory systems are not comprehensive or mature like those of western countries. India does not dedicate enough resources to medical malpractice lawsuits, and its Medical Council Act is "outdated and ineffective." Most foreign insurance companies do not recognize Indian medical qualifications. And as recently as 2001, India had a net loss of patients—the number of patients that left India for medical treatment exceeded the number of foreign patients that visited. Thus, while India is quickly becoming a leading destination for patients, its health sector lags.

Malaysia

In 2002 and 2003, Malaysian hospitals treated 103,000 foreign patients, 75,000 of whom visited specifically for health care. Patients travelled from Indonesia, India, the Middle East, and the United Kingdom seeking treatments in cardiology, haematology, gastroenterology, neurology, and cosmetic surgery. The government has aggressively courted foreign patients, creating a National Committee for medical tourism in 1998, which is headed by the Minister for Culture, Arts, and Tourism. The National Economic Action Council hopes to make Malaysia "a worldclass regional health care centre." The government's "Eighth Malaysia Plan" selected thirty-five private hospitals to market overseas and called for public hospitals to create private wings for foreign patients.

Singapore

Singapore treated roughly 200,000 foreign patients in 2003, 10% of whom visited specifically for medical care. Patients visit from Asia, Australia, the United Kingdom, and the United States, seeking treatments in general surgery, cardiac surgery, ophthalmology, orthopedic surgery, gynecology, and urology. Singapore helped pioneer medical tourism in Asia, but providers there have felt increasing competition from other countries. In response, the Ministry of Health called for efforts to retain Singapore's status as the "healthcare hub of Asia." An official report recommended supporting more clinical research, recruiting of health care professionals, and cooperation between public and private providers, as well as easing advertising restrictions and dedicating an agency to coordinate these efforts. The government established Singapore Medicine, which represents the Ministry of Health, the Singapore Tourism Board, and other key agencies. Singapore's Tourism Board also established the Healthcare Services Strategic Tourism Unit in 2003 to promote local hospitals, establish referral channels overseas, and help implement an accreditation system. Singapore's goal is to treat one million foreign patients per year by 2012. Singapore's model is one developing countries may try to emulate, particularly the creation of a centralized, public-private partnership to coordinate industry efforts.

Thailand

In 2002 and 2003 Thailand treated nearly 630,000 foreign patients, 126,000 of whom visited specifically for health care. Along with Singapore, Thailand helped pioneer medical tourism in Asia. Patients visit primarily from Southeast Asia, Europe, and the United States, seeking treatments in cardiac surgery, cosmetic surgery, dentistry, cataract surgery, and bone-related procedures. In the late 1990s, the Tourism Authority began a campaign that included medical tourism. The government now plans to spend nearly $3 million to advertise and develop health care centres in Bangkok, Phuket, and Chiang Mai. Thailand also has very permissive visa policies, which either do not require visas or provide them on arrival to citizens of over 150 countries.

United Kingdom

The United Kingdom's experience reveals the multifarious nature of medical tourism. On one hand, U.K. citizens travel overseas to bypass long waiting lists, and the National Health Service (NHS) sends patients on waiting lists to other EU countries for certain surgeries. On the other hand, the United Kingdom is also a major destination for foreign patients, which has stretched waiting lists and NHS resources. Foreign citizens currently occupy 20% of hospital beds in London. The United Kingdom has reciprocal arrangements with sixty countries to provide the same medical care to foreign nationals as they do to local citizens. Regulations require the NHS to charge for health care provided to anyone who is "not ordinarily [a] resident in the U.K.," but many believe loopholes in these regulations are being abused. The public has scrutinized foreign citizens who are exempt from being charged by the NHS, particularly business travellers who schedule treatments in U.K. hospitals. The NHS has considered various ways to discourage medical tourists from visiting, for example, by asking patients to confirm their residency and creating a mandatory NHS patient card. Critics have even proposed withdrawing free nonemergency care for asylum seekers whose asylum applications have been denied. The United Kingdom's struggle with medical tourism reflects both the challenges developing countries face in allocating scarce resources between local and foreign patients, and the challenges developed countries face in dealing with jurisdictional boundaries.

United States

Much like the United Kingdom, the United States both imports and exports patients. For decades, the United States has attracted wealthy foreign patients for the advanced, specialized medical care offered here. At the same time, the National Coalition on Health Care estimated that nearly 500,000 U.S. patients travelled overseas in 2005.

Chile

Chile has become a regional medical hub in Latin America, attracting patients from Bolivia, Peru, and Ecuador. Chile has targeted Bolivian patients through private insurers and national health care centres. Chilean clinics have established agreements with Bolivian health care centres to treat Bolivian patients.

Cuba

Since the 1980s, Cuba has made a concentrated effort to become a "world medical power." It hosts a significant number of patients from Latin America, the Caribbean, Russia, and the United Kingdom, who generally seek niche procedures in ophthalmology, joint surgery, neurology, and treatments for skin diseases. The government created the company Servimed to arrange medical treatments and travel for foreign patients. The government has also signed bilateral agreements with Latin American and Caribbean governments to facilitate medical tourism, with the parties even negotiating prices. Finally, Cuba provides free or subsidized care to patients from certain countries.

Jordan

Jordan treated 70,000 foreign patients in 2002 and 2003, primarily from the Middle East. Jordanian hospitals specialize in cardiac surgery, spinal injuries, cornea transplants, and alternative medicine. Since the early 1990s, Jordan has tried to become the medical hub for the Arab world. The government has created incentives for private investment in the health sector, which has generated several new private hospitals. The public sector has also modernized its hospitals and medical schools, some of which are electronically linked with prestigious hospitals in Europe and North America.

Other Countries

The nine countries above are the most notable players in the global patient market, but several others are seeking to attract foreign patients, including Argentina, China, Colombia, Costa Rica, the Dominican Republic, the Philippines, and South Africa. Mexico has long attracted U.S. patients seeking dental care, access to affordable pharmaceuticals, and cosmetic surgeries. And after being admitted into the European Community, Turkey has quickly become a medical tourist destination, with low costs and a profusion of JCI-accredited hospitals. Thus, even in its relatively infant stages, medical tourism represents a diverse set of countries, medical procedures, and export strategies.

Analysing the Risks and Opportunities in Medical Tourism

The following paragraphs examines the risks and opportunities by analysing how it may affect health care costs, quality, and access in the United States and in developing countries. Several scholars identify these three canonical themes as the core framework for analysing health care issues.

Costs and Financing

The recent wave of medical tourism is being driven by cost discrepancies. Treatments in developing countries are documented to be 50–90% less expensive than in the United States. For example, inpatient knee surgery may cost an average of $10,335 in the United States versus $1236 at many foreign hospitals. Hysterectomies cost $5783 in the United States versus $1869 in developing countries. The disparities are more pronounced with complex, expensive procedures. A coronary artery bypass graft may cost $60,000 in the United States versus $10,000 or less in India. A bone marrow transplant may cost $250,000 in the United States versus $30,000 in India or $60,000 in Thailand.

Such cost discrepancies may tempt U.S. employers and insurers to explore the use of foreign providers. After all, health care spending continues to perplex the United States. US spend far more on health care than any other country, but the citizen are neither healthier nor happier with the system. In a 2006 Senate hearing on medical tourism, Senator Gordon Smith opined that "Americans should not have to travel overseas to obtain affordable health care." But in a system looking for any way to relieve the intense cost pressures, medical tourism seems to be a logical release valve. Senator Smith acknowledged that "[f]or the nation's 46 million uninsured, travelling overseas for low-cost medical procedures, even with the added cost of travel and lodging, is an understandably attractive option." This section examines how medical tourism may impact health spending in the United States and in developing countries.

Health Insurance

Few public or private U.S. insurers cover nonemergency medical care overseas. Medicare and Medicaid only pay for treatment overseas under narrow circumstances. For example, Medicare covers nonemergency services overseas only if the hospital is more accessible from the beneficiary's residence than any suitable U.S. hospital. Thus, if a Medicare beneficiary living in Guam needs treatment, and the nearest adequate hospital is in the Philippines, federal law permits Medicare to pay for the services in the Philippines. Otherwise, Medicare coverage is non-portable.

Private insurance is slightly more portable, but most private insurers also cover only emergency services overseas. The World Bank found that most U.S. managed care organizations cover only emergency services overseas, treating it as an out-of-network benefit, which requires patients to spend more out-of-pocket. Some plans require the patient to pay for the entire treatment upfront and seek reimbursement after returning to the United States. Virtually no insurers cover travel expenses, which effectively makes insurance even less portable. The World Bank study found these to be significant market barriers.

Nevertheless, there are two significant examples of governments paying for nonemergency medical care overseas: the EU and TRICARE. First, since the 1970s, EU regulations have required member states to reimburse their citizens for medical care they receive in other states in certain circumstances, for example, when the citizen needs emergency care or when the citizen cannot obtain the treatment where she resides in a medically appropriate timeframe. Recently, a series of court cases has eroded the authority of member states to require prior authorization or deny reimbursement for medical treatments in other EU countries. The cases together generally hold that Articles 49 and 50 of the European Community Treaty which prohibit member states from restricting the free movement of persons and services throughout the EU—trump the authority of states to administer their own health insurance systems. The European Court of Justice has interpreted these articles very broadly to invalidate a wide variety of national rules. Previously, many states interpreted the EU regulations narrowly, rarely granting prior authorization. Thus, although member states still retain the authority to decide when their citizens will be reimbursed for medical care in other EU states, they must make their national health insurance more portable within the EU. Most EU states now reimburse patients for travel and living expenses when treated abroad, and some states cover the expenses of a travel companion.

Second, the U.S. government covers medical care overseas for military personnel and their dependants through TRICARE, the Department of Defense's managed care program. The TRICARE Overseas Program enrolls beneficiaries, processes claims, contracts with foreign providers, and certifies foreign providers for acceptance into its "Preferred Provider Network." Moreover, TRICARE uses regional "Health Care Finders" to locate referrals for specialty care, authorize certain treatments, and assist beneficiaries.

Thus, although health insurance is generally non-portable, TRICARE and the EU show how portable insurance is likely to look in practice. United States health insurers can look to these programs for examples of how to establish a network of foreign providers, process foreign claims, and monitor foreign providers.

Gains from Trade

A World Bank economist found that the price differences between the United States and developing countries should create "a strong incentive for trade." To estimate the gains from trade, the authors selected fifteen surgeries that were "highly tradable," that is, surgeries that are low-risk, nonemergency treatments with quick recovery periods. Factoring in travel costs, the authors found that the United States could save $1.4 billion annually if only ten percent of patients travelled overseas for these procedures. Roughly half of these savings ($690 million) would accrue to Medicare. By adding coronary artery bypass grafts to the list of "highly tradable" procedures, annual savings would then exceed $2 billion.

The authors acknowledge that $2 billion is a small portion of U.S. health care spending. It is unclear whether the market will grow enough to significantly affect U.S. health care prices. Two experts note that "non-urgent surgeries that are costly enough to offset travel costs and required incentives [to travel overseas] account for less than two percent of commercial insurance spending." However, the World Bank authors explain that the savings could be much larger. The $2 billion savings estimate included only fifteen procedures, though patients travel for many more. The study also used Medicare payment rates to calculate U.S. prices, "which are lower than those paid by private insurers and the uninsured." Finally, the authors did not have patient volume data for certain procedures, which may further underestimate the savings.

The World Bank made no parallel estimate of how much developing countries stand to gain from medical tourism, but other sources show the gains to be significant. Barely ten years ago, Cuba was already generating $25 million per year from medical tourism. Malaysia earned $103 million in 2003 and aims to increase revenue tenfold by 2010. India may soon generate over $2 billion per year from medical tourism. An optimistic observer predicts that by 2010, medical tourism will generate $40 billion per year. These revenues may allow developing countries to upgrade their medical schools, facilities, technology, and overall health care infrastructure. Moreover, the additional foreign money could significantly reduce the burden on government health care spending if the revenues are appropriately directed. Thus, medical tourism may have a material financial impact in the United States and in developing countries.

Cross-Border Health Insurance

As the gains from trade become apparent and as U.S. health care spending continues to rise, more insurers will consider using offshore providers. Some insurers have already made the leap. Three insurers in California pay for U.S. residents to obtain medical care in Mexico. Health Net offers plans to employers and individuals under its "Salud con Health Net" program. The Mexican insurer SIMNSA offers similar plans, sometimes in conjunction with Health Net. BlueShield offers "Access Baja" to its customers who live near the border. These plans generally offer lower premiums and deductibles than plans that pay only for U.S. providers.

Other insurers are stretching well beyond Mexico. United Group Programs recently added the Bumrungrad Hospital in Thailand to its preferred provider network. Blue Cross Blue Shield and the British insurer Bupa insure patients treated at the Wockhardt Hospitals in India. In fact, Blue Cross Blue Shield helps its members obtain emergency and nonemergency care overseas through its BlueCard Worldwide program, which is run by a company that maintains a global network of hospitals, physicians, and other health care providers.

Public insurers are also looking overseas. In 2006, West Virginia legislators proposed a bill that would give state public employees incentives to seek medical treatments overseas at JCI-accredited hospitals. The bill asks the state to:

— waive copayments and deductibles,
— pay the round-trip airfare and up to seven days of hotel expenses for the employee and one companion,
— compensate the employer for sick leave, and
— pay up to twenty percent of the cost savings to the employee.

The proposal would deposit the remaining eighty percent of cost savings into a state fund, with rebates distributed to employees covered under West Virginia's Public Employees Insurance Agency. The legislators intended the bill to encourage competition among West Virginia providers.

Foreign providers are also contacting U.S. insurers. Private clinics in Canada are contacting U.S. insurers to offer medical services at a fraction of U.S. prices. The Apollo Group in India is negotiating with insurers in the United States and Europe to design ways to encourage patients to visit India for certain elective procedures. Several hospitals also have in-house departments that liaise with foreign insurers.

Thus, health insurance is becoming more portable. EU member states cover treatments abroad out of legal necessity. TRICARE covers treatments abroad out of practical necessity. And Californian insurers cover treatments in Mexico out of demographic necessity insuring a population that traditionally lacks health insurance and may prefer Spanish-speaking providers. These early adopters may be setting a precedent for other U.S. insurers, as some mainstream insurers are now considering foreign providers primarily for cost-saving reasons.

Moral Hazards

Paying for medical care overseas is not without risk. Cross-border insurers face the same problems that confront domestic insurers, such as fraud, abuse, and moral hazard (the threat that the insured will overconsume health care precisely because they are insured). Moreover, these problems may be magnified when dealing with foreign providers that operate under different legal, regulatory, and financial systems.

Nevertheless, the World Bank proposed using traditional insurance tools to combat these problems. To combat fraud and abuse by foreign providers such as overbilling and providing unnecessary treatments insurers can require utilization reviews by which U.S. physicians can verify the need for treatment *ex ante,* and the receipt of treatment *ex post.* Insurers can also create international provider networks to monitor foreign providers. The threat of being removed from a provider network and losing access to the lucrative U.S. market would give providers a strong incentive to avoid allegations of fraud. Finally, insurers can sign contracts with foreign providers that grant insurers audit rights, increasing transparency.

To minimize moral hazard, the World Bank authors state that insurers can create cross-border plans with lower premiums and higher deductibles. The lower premiums could encourage patients to travel abroad in the first instance patients that do not wish to travel abroad could choose domestic plans with higher premiums and the higher deductibles could discourage moral hazard. Indeed, some insurers in California already use lower premiums to encourage California residents to visit Mexican providers, and as the World Bank authors note, private insurers use different premiums and deductibles for out-of-network providers. Creating cross-border plans is merely an extension of that practice.

It is not clear whether we should be as optimistic as the World Bank that traditional insurance tools can effectively mitigate fraud, abuse, and moral hazard in overseas medical care, as these tools have arguably not worked well in the United States. Nevertheless, combining these tools with international provider networks and other incentive structures may make cross-border health insurance more plausible.

General Concerns

Medical tourism raises quality concerns because patients must travel both before and after treatment. Patients may not receive adequate pre-screening from foreign providers. Although the top foreign hospitals often facilitate contact between physicians and foreign patients, these contacts generally are remote. Physicians can review medical histories, test results, and even communicate with patients, but they cannot physically examine the patient until he or she arrives, which may be only days before surgery. Thus, the pre-screening process may not adequately replicate the in-person screening process that . physicians perform.

Physicians also worry that patients may not receive adequate postoperative care overseas. Patients may underestimate their recovery times when booking travel arrangements. Even patients who take time to convalesce may have difficulty obtaining checkups or follow-up procedures. Physicians may be reluctant to provide follow-up care for surgeries performed overseas. Insurers fear that patients will return with complications, and insurers may not cover remedial care. Finally, the uninsured medical tourist who pays for the procedure out-of-pocket may not be able to afford follow-up treatments in the United States.

One possible solution is for insurers and hospitals to use international provider networks to pre-screen patients and to provide follow-up care in the United States. Global hospital networks like the Apollo Group and Adventist Health International may already take advantage of their international networks. Indeed, Penang Adventist Hospital reportedly instructs patients who experience complications to visit one of its affiliate hospitals in the United States and "not worry about money." Although this claim seems dubious, international provider networks can reduce the risks that patients will not receive adequate pre-screening or postoperative care. Insurers can even adopt a hybrid approach by outsourcing expensive surgeries while performing pre-screening and follow-up care in the United States.

Regulatory Disincentives

Another structural feature of medical tourism that raises quality concerns is the risk that global competition will create perverse regulatory disincentives. As medical tourism becomes more lucrative, countries may compete by offering treatments that other countries do not offer. Poor countries may be tempted to offer treatments that are illegal or highly experimental elsewhere. One author worries that competition for patients in Asia may encourage poorer countries like Cambodia, Laos, and Myanmar to "engage in less reputable practices that are illegal or not widely obtainable." This competitive dynamic is particularly striking with controversial practices, such as organ transplantations and xenotransplantations. For example, patients seeking xenotransplantation procedures visit countries like Mexico for controversial treatments that can be exceedingly dangerous.

Competition for patients may recreate the same regulatory "race to the bottom" that has affected other global markets. Governments may be reluctant to place legal restrictions on local businesses that may raise prices or otherwise hamper their ability to compete.

Some patients will always vote with their feet and travel to countries with more permissive laws. When patients leave the United States, they are expressing a distinct policy preference for a foreign system even if the expression is temporary. For example, U.S. patients travelled to Europe, Asia, and India for a hip resurfacing procedure that was not approved by the FDA until recently. Reproductive tourists are particularly assertive forum shoppers. In 2001, after the FDA began banning several controversial fertility treatments, couples began travelling overseas for the procedures. Patients are more willing than ever to leave the United States if they are not satisfied with the procedures available here. At the same time, such patients are taking a calculated risk. Horror stories abound of patients being seriously injured from cosmetic surgeries in developing countries. The media frequently reports new incidents in which medical tourists have returned home with complications from failed procedures.

Patients may frustrate domestic regulators by travelling overseas for controversial or experimental treatments. Medical tourism may thwart the FDA's efforts to regulate a particular treatment or technology, and may also profoundly affect domestic research and development. Companies seeking FDA approval for products increasingly rely on data from clinical trials in developing countries, particularly when they are under financial and time pressures to complete studies.

Patient Autonomy

Medical tourists exercise autonomy by seeking medical treatments in other jurisdictions not for cost reasons, but because the treatments are banned by law or regulation where they live. This happens most often with fertility treatments, and it has generated some debate. The concern is that medical tourism allows patients to buy their way out of restrictive local laws and regulations. As travel becomes less expensive, some wonder whether "any single jurisdiction can continue to enforce its own rules." Guido Pennings argues that international travel has made it "impossible to enforce laws that people do not consider morally justified." Thus, he argues that legislating medical treatments will be primarily a symbolic public statement of the majority's moral convictions. As an example, Pennings points to the

Swiss Federal Council, which lobbied against a law that would have banned most forms of *in vitro* fertilization because the law would merely encourage infertile couples to travel overseas. In effect, such laws may remove the government's control over controversial medical procedures, forcing governments to confront their limited jurisdiction. Is it fair that laws and regulations apply only to patients that cannot afford to choose another system? Are medical tourists breaching or at least opting out of a social contract with our health care system? Are these dangers worth the increased autonomy for patients?

There are compelling arguments both ways. The strongest argument for medical tourism is that it is equally unfair to deny access to treatments that are available in other countries. Some in the European Union argue that it would be unfair for a member state to deny its citizens access to medical services that other EU citizens can obtain. In fact, the remedies may be worse than the problem. Some EU countries have used extremely draconian methods to restrict reproductive tourism, and there are real legal and practical limits to denying U.S. patients access to foreign treatments as well.

A related argument is that medical tourism allows patients to exercise autonomy and "vote with their feet." In modern societies characterized by diverging viewpoints, medical tourism may be a "pragmatic solution to the problem of how to combine the democratic system which proceeds according to majority rule, with a degree of individual freedom for members of the minority." Allowing patients to vote with their feet may alleviate the "tyranny of the majority" that expresses itself through laws and regulations. This argument requires us to accept a degree of moral pluralism some citizens may simply prefer medical care in a country with policies that more closely align with their personal moral judgments.

However, if patients can vote with their feet, they may lose interest in reforming their own health care system. When voters disagree with policies, they can change them through the cumbersome democratic process or simply leave the jurisdiction. In many cases, it takes less effort to simply leave. For example, if Congress bans a certain fertility treatment, infertile couples may travel overseas rather than fight to repeal the law. Although a patient exodus may cause the government to reconsider its policies, some governments may be content to see the problem exported overseas.

References

Bartha M. Knoppers & Sonia LeBris, (1991). Recent Advances in Medically Assisted Conception: Legal, Ethical, and Social Issues, 17 *Am. J.l.&Med.* 329, 333.

Diana M. Ernst, (Sept. 2006). Medical Tourism: Why Americans Take Medical Vacations Abroad, 4 *Pac. Res. Inst.* 1.

Edwin Borman, (2004). Health Tourism: Where Healthcare, Ethics, and the State Collide, 328 *Brit. Med. J.* 60, 60.

Ganapati Mudur, (2004). Hospitals in India Woo Foreign Patients, 328 *Brit. Med. J.* 1338, 1338.

Johanna Paola D. Poblete, (2007). Special Feature: Medical Tourism, *Bus. World*, Philippines.

Linda F. Powers, (2006). Leveraging Medical Tourism, *The Scientist*, March

Nicolas P. Terry, (2007), Under-Regulated Healthcare Phenomena in a Flat World: Medical Tourism and Outsourcing, 29 *W. New Eng. L. Rev.* 421 .

5

Trends in Indian Medical Tourism Industry

India is the land of myriad experiences and exotic locales. It is a world of resplendent colours and rich cultural locales, be it magnificent monuments, heritage temples or tombs. The Country's ancient cultural heritage is inextricably linked to its technology driven present existence. The co-existence of a number of religions and cultures, together with an awe-inspiring topography makes it the perfect place for a complete holiday experience. The Indian medical tourism industry, growing at an annual rate of 30 percent, caters to patients chiefly from the US, Europe, West Asia and Africa. Although in its nascent stage, the industry is outsmarting similar industries of other countries such as Greece, South Africa, Jordan, Malaysia, Philippines and Singapore. In 2006, over 1,50,000 medical tourists have visited India and is growing by 15% a year. The medical tourism industry in India is presently earning revenues of $450 million . Encouraged by the incredible pace of growth exhibited by the industry, the Confederation of Indian Industry (CII) and McKinsey have predicted that the industry will grow to earn additional revenue of $2.2 billion by 2012. India, touted as the favourite destination for information technology majors, is currently emerging as a preferred destination for medical or health tourism.

The Government of India, State tourism boards, travel agents, tour operators, hotel companies and private sector hospitals are exploring the medical tourism industry for tremendous opportunities. They are seeking to capitalize on the opportunities by combining the country's popular leisure tourism with medical tourism. The factors that make India as one of the favorable destination for health tourism starts with low medical cost which is one-tenth of the costs in western countries, for example, a heart surgery costs $ 6,000 in India as against $30,000 in the US, Similarly a bone marrow transplant costs $26,000 in India as compared to $2, 50,000 in the US. Foreign patients throng Indian hospitals to pass up the long waiting lists and queues in their native countries.Globalization has promoted a consumerist culture, thereby promoting goods and services that can feed the aspirations arising from this culture. This has had its effect in the health sector too. There are number of reasons for the growth of the service economy and these can be categorized into three main areas such as:

1. Social trend
2. Demographic trends
3. New services to meet new demands

The new services to meet new demand may include the "medical tourism". Merging healthcare and tourism an industry has been evolved in many developing countries like Greece, South Africa, Jordan, India, Malaysia, Philippines and Singapore. Medical tourism where foreigners travel abroad in search of low cost, world-class medical treatment is gaining popularity in India. India's medical tourism industry could yield as much as $3 billion in annual revenue by 2012. Indian government hopes to encourage a budding trade in medical tourism, selling foreigners the idea of traveling to India for low cost but world class medical treatment.

According to the confederation of Indian industry India has the potential to attract 1 million tourists per annum, which could contribute to $6 billion to the economy. India must leverage its competitive edge, especially its cost advantage. It is only one fifth of the costs in the west. Cost savings may not be enough to foster a trade in medical tourism. Unfairly or not, most foreigners would not think of India as a land of good health. The sight of the countries overcrowded public hospitals; open sewers and garbage littered streets would unsettle most visitors' confidence about public sanitation standards in India. Private healthcare providers argue that foreigners can be sheltered from such nastiness and that the qualities of India's corporate hospitals are world class.

Currently medical tourists or medical travelers from developed industrialized countries are traveling in large numbers abroad where the quality of healthcare is equal to or even better than the standards in their own country and yet the cost is significantly lower. These healthcare destination countries also offer numerous options for escapes to vacation touring trips, sight-seeing, shopping, exploring journeys and lounging on sun drenched exotic beaches for medical health care travelers. A combination of many factors has lead to the recent increase in the popularity of medical tourism or Medical value travel. Exorbitant cost of basic health care and medical insurance cover, high cost of modern medical facilities in advanced countries, ease and affordability of international travel, favorable currency exchange rates in the global economy, rapidly improving technology and high standards of medical care in the developing countries, best medical health care education at the medical schools, proven safety of healthcare in select foreign nations, international accreditation of foreign hospitals and access to U.S., U.K. and Australian board certified surgeons operating in select foreign countries have all contributed their share to this rapid development of global medical tourism or medical health care outsourcing.

Health care tourism or medical health care value travel has also emerged as a most popular form of vacationing mixing a broad spectrum of overseas medical health care services with leisure, a visit to health care resort or a health SPA abroad, fun and relaxation together thereby maximizing the value of vacation travel abroad, a holiday retreat with wellness and health care. Most of the foreigners treated in India come from other developing countries in Asia, Africa or the middle east where top quality hospitals and health professionals are often hard to find. Patients from the United States and Europe are relatively rare not only because of the distance they must travel but also hospital executives acknowledge because India continues to suffer from an image of poverty and poor hygiene that discourages many patients.

Market for Medical Tourism

India has always been a regional health care hub for the health care tourists from the neighboring countries like Afghanistan, Bangladesh,

Pakistan, Nepal, Bhutan, UAE and Maldives; recently India has emerged as one of the most important Global destination for medical tourism or health care travel. Now international patients from the developed countries like USA, Canada, UK, Europe etc. travel to India for the low-cost medical surgery treatments like knee joint replacement, total hip replacement, hip resurfacing, weight loss procedures- gastric lap band, RNY gastric bypass, heart procedures, elective surgeries and also for rejuvenation therapies promised by yoga and Ayurveda. However, a nice blend of top-class medical expertise at attractive prices is helping more and more corporate hospitals in India to lure global foreign patients for high end surgeries like organ transplants.

As more and more patients from Europe, North America and other affluent nations with very high medical costs and long wait lists look for effective options of immediate, low-cost, affordable treatments, medical health care travel to India is definitely on the cards for most of them and the fast growing Indian corporate health sector is fully geared to meet that need. Medical tourism to India is not just cost savings or the high standard of medical care facility, but also the waiting time for medical surgery treatment procedures in India is much lower than in any other country.

India offers a growing number of private centers of excellence where the quality of care is as good as or better than that of big-city hospitals in the United States or Europe. The medical care sector in India has witnessed an enormous growth in infrastructure in the private and voluntary sector. The private sector, which was very modest in the early stages, has now becoming a flourishing industry equipped with the most modern state of the art technology at its disposal. It is estimated that 75% of healthcare services and investments in India are now provided by the private sector. Health and medical tourism is perceived as one of the fastest growing segments in marketing destination India today. India could earn $2 billion annually and create 60 million new jobs by subcontracting work from the British National Health Service, the head of India's largest chain of private hospitals.

Medical tourism is growing and diversifying. Estimates vary, but McKinsey & Company and the Confederation of Indian Industry put gross medical tourism revenues at more than $40 billion worldwide in 2004. Others estimate the worldwide revenue at about $60 billion in

2006. McKinsey & Company projects the total will rise to $100 billion by 2012.

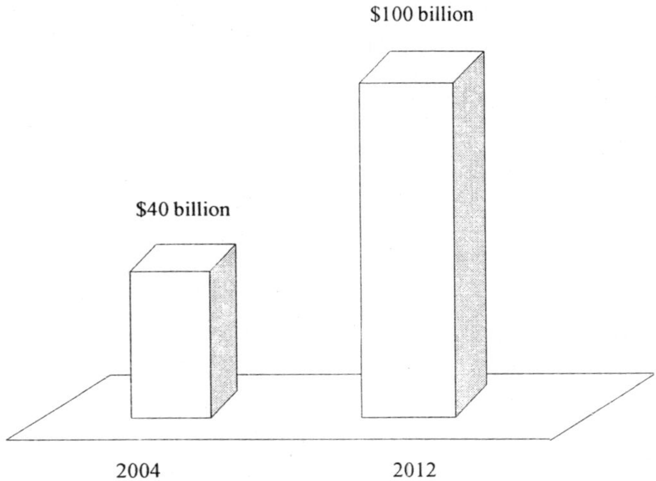

Figure 1. World wide medical tourism Indutsry (in billions of Us dollars)

According to the confederation of Indian Industry India has the potential to attract 2 million tourist per annum which could contribute to $ 5 billion to the economy. India must leverage its competitive edge especially cost advantage. It is only one fifth of the cost in the west. India enjoys a unique position as it offers holistic medicinal services. With yoga, meditation, ayurveda, allopathic and other systems of medicines, India offers a unique basket of services to an individual that is difficult to match by other countries. Also, clinical outcomes in India are at par with the world's best centers besides having internationally qualified and experienced specialists. The equation in India to promote the industry is first world treatment at third world prices. A CII – McKinsey report last year, postulating the opportunities in health tourism industry states that the medical tourism market in the country pegged a 30 percent growth in 2000 and it has been growing at the rate of 15 percent for the past five years. The report says by 2012, if medical tourism were to reach 25 percent revenues of private up market players up to Rs.10000 crore will be added to the revenues of these players.

SCOPE OF MEDICAL TOURISM IN INDIA

The main demand for medical tou.ism is generated from millions of Indians who live abroad, though a growing number of foreigners are also keen on speedy and in expensive treatment. They are influenced by two important facts: India now has many world-class private hospitals and Indian doctors have experience in abundance. Owing to India's prodigious population, the strengths in health care sector is doctors treat twice the number of patients in comparison to doctors in the west, domestic aviation has been opened to the private sector, foreign investments are encouraged and a number of incentives are in place. India is considered as a safe destination compared to other countries Foreigners are visiting India for serious medical help as well as rejuvenation therapies and other specific purposes.

Medical tourism is poised to be the next Indian success story after Information Technology. According to recent study the industry's earning potential estimated at Rs.5000-10000 crores by2012. The main reason for India emerging as a referred destination is the inherent advantage of its health care industry. India offers a variety of services for overseas patients. Generation of foreign exchange, creation of income, generation of employment, contribution to state revenue and its associated regional development can be cited as the major economic benefits of tourism. The demand for Indian health care services primarily comes from three types of consumers

i) Non-Residential Indians

ii) Patients from countries with underdeveloped facilities

iii) Patients from developed countries.

Though tourism is not the primary need of these consumers, it offers additional attraction particularly for people travelling for cosmetic surgery and less complicated procedures.

India's health care sector is on the road to global fame. India is the seat of spiritualism. It is the confluence of different religions: Hinduism, Sikhism, Christianity, Islam and Jainism etc. Medical tourism in India is promoted as high-tech healing destinations, which provide world-class treatment at low cost, incorporating the Indian Systems of Medicine. India offers world-class treatments and a leisure holiday at excellent locations at almost 50 percent less than the total sum the foreign patients would spent on treatment in their own country. Foreigners are attracted to Indian Systems of Medicine (ISM) and tourism. The Indian Systems of Medicine include Ayurveda, Yoga and Naturopathy, Unani, Siddha and Homoeopathy together characterized under the department of AYUSH in the union health and family welfare ministry. During the ninth plan, with an expenditure of more than Rs.1,000 crore, a quantum jump in outlays on schemes for development and promotion of AYUSH system of medicine has been achieved during Tenth Plan.

Indians are known for their hospitality and warmth.India has an incomparibly rich heritage in ancient systems of medicine that make up a veritable treasure house of knowledge for both preventive and curative health care. Around 1000 BC when Indian Systems of Medicine (ISM) were fully documented in Charaka Samhita and Sushruta Samhita. Thus, ISM is considered to be one of the oldest organized systems of medicine for positive health and cure of human sickness. The most important and massive ancient compilation of the school of medicine is known as Charaka Samhita. It contains several chapters dealing at length with internal medicine. About six hundred drugs of plant, animal and mineral origin are described in it. So far so good. But traditional medicine was ignored when western medical knowledge and procedures were introduced into the country.

Ayurveda : Ayurveda means the "science of life" in Sanskrit. It is one of oldest and the best documented among the ancient systems of medicine. From the Charaka Samhita (600 B.C) and the Susruta samhita.

Yoga: Yoga is not really a system of medicine. Its objectives are self- realization and spiritual union with all –pervasive divine cosmic power. But certain intermediary practices and yogic attitudes have proved beneficial for reducing stress, preventing many lifestyle-related diseases, and promoting general health and well being.

Naturopathy: Naturopathy is based on the fundamental principles of ayurveda. The basic tenet of Naturopathy is to live according to the laws of nature: disease occurs due to the accumulation of toxins in the body, and to cure the ailment, the body is purified with the use of natural methods, dietary regulations and exercise.

Unani :The Unani system originated in the fourth and fifth century BC in Greece under the patronage of Hippocrates (460BC-377)and Galen. The system is based on the humoural theory that good health depends on the balance of the four humours: blood, phlegm, yellow bile and black bile.

Siddha : Siddha means a "master" thus the name denoted the mastery of such practices. The most famous of the siddha was Nagarjuna, whose rasatantra forms the basis of this system. The distinctive features of siddha are its reliance on minerals and metallic compounds, and its emphasis on rejuvenation therapies.

Homeopathy: The term homeopathy comes from the Greek word 'homios' means like and 'pathos' means suffering. Homeopathyworks by looking at the symptoms, will take into account the individual's mental, physical, emotional,and spiritual health before deciding the treatment. Homeopathy is based on the principles that 'like cures like'.

Due to liberlisation of our economy and internalization of health care profession, India has entered the industry in only recent times. India's corporate hospitals are fully equipped with up market and efficiency. With their toll free lines, interactive websites, online quotes and time bound treatment access, they appear to be a world apart from the over burden, often badly managed and poorly funded public health system.

There is no doubt that the Indian medical industry's main appeal is low cost treatment. Most estimates claim treatment costs in India start around a tenth of the price of comparable treatment in leading countries of the world. AIIMS is a destination for patients from Nepal, Bangladesh, Bhutan, Myanmar, Mauritius and Pakistan. Besides regular patients from the Middle East, and an occasional patient drop from US and other European countries. Patients from Pakistan, especially children with heart affiliation, have been regularly coming to ai India medical science. When baby Noor Fatima, a two and a half year old Pakistani girl, successfully underwent an open heart surgery in India, she opened news vistas reminding the potential of medical tourism. In 2003 the number of patients who visited the hospital was 5000 and about 1500 was hospitalized. Along with providing treatment, the stay of the foreign patients is taken care of by the hospital itself. CII along with IHCF is working with tour operators to promote attractive packages for medical tourism.

The Indian government predicts that India's $20 billion a year health-care industry could grow 13 percent in each of the next six years, boosted by medical tourism, which industry watchers say is growing at 35 percent annually. In India, the Apollo group alone has so far treated 100000 international patients, many of whom are of Indian origin Apollo has been a forerunner in medical tourism in India and attracts patients from Southeast Asia, Africa and the Middle East. The group has tied up with hospitals in Mauritius, Tanzania, Bangladesh and Yemen besides running a hospital in srilanka and managing a hospital in Dubai.

Another corporate group running a chain of hospitals, escorts claims it has doubled its number of overseas patients from 1000 in 2000 to 3000 this year. In India the strong tradition of traditional systems of healthcare in kerala, for example is utilized. Kerala Ayurveda centers have been established at multiple locations in various metro cities, thus highlighting the advantages of ayurveda in health management.

The countries where medical tourism is being actively promoted include Greece, South Africa, Jordan, India, Malaysia, Philippines and Singapore. India is a recent entrant into medical tourism. According to a study by McKinsey and the Confederation of Indian Industry, medical tourism in India could become a $1 billion business by 2012. The report predicts that: "By 2012, if medical tourism were to reach 25 per cent of revenues of private up-market players, up to Rs 10,000 crore will be added to the revenues of these players".

Cost-effectiveness of Indian Medical Tourism

The key "selling points" of the medical tourism industry are its "cost effectiveness" and its combination with the attractions of tourism. The latter also uses the ploy of selling the "exotica" of the countries involved as well as the packaging of health care with traditional therapies and treatment methods. Price advantage is, of course, a major selling point. The slogan, thus is, "First World treatment' at Third World prices". The cost differential across the board is huge: only a tenth and sometimes even a sixteenth of the cost in the West. Open-heart surgery could cost up to $70,000 in Britain and up to $150,000 in the US; in India's best hospitals it could cost between $3,000 and $10,000. Knee surgery (on both knees) costs 350,000 rupees ($7,700) in India; in Britain this costs £10,000 ($16,950), more than twice as much. Dental, eye and cosmetic surgeries in Western countries cost three to four times as much as in India. The price advantage is however offset today for patients from the developed countries by concerns regarding standards, insurance coverage and other infrastructure. This is where the tourism and medical industries are trying to pool resources, and also putting pressure on the government. We shall turn to their implications later. In India the strong tradition of traditional systems of health care in Kerala, for example, is utilized. Kerala Ayurveda centres have been established at multiple locations in various metro cities, thus highlighting the advantages of Ayurveda in health management.

Table 1. Comparing the Costs of Dental care India with USA

Dental procedure	*Cost in USA ($)*		*Cost in India ($)*
	General Dentist	*Top End Dentist*	*Top End Dentist*
Smile designing	-	8,000	1,000
Metal Free Bridge	-	5,500	500
Dental Implants	-	3,500	800
Porcelain Metal Bridge	1,800	3,000	300
Porcelain Metal Crown	600	1,000	80
Tooth impactions	500	2,000	100
Root canal Treatment	600	1,000	100
Tooth whitening	350	800	110
Tooth colored composite	200	500	25
Tooth cleaning	100	300	75

The health tourism focus has seen Kerala participate in various trade shows and expos wherein the advantages of this traditional form of medicine are showcased. A generic problem with medical tourism is that it reinforces the medicalised view of health care. By promoting the notion that medical services can be bought off the shelf from the lowest priced provider anywhere in the globe, it also takes away the pressure from the government to provide comprehensive health care to all its citizens. It is a deepening of the whole notion of health care that is being pushed today which emphasizes on technology and private enterprise.

Table 2. Medical Procedure Charges in India & USA

Procedure	*United States (USD) Approx*	*India (USD) Approx*
Bone Marrow Transplant	USD 2,50,000	USD 69,200
Liver Transplant	USD 3,00,000	USD 69,350
Heart Surgery	USD 30,000	USD 8,700
Orthopedic Surgery	USD 20,000	USD 6,300
Cataract Surgery	USD 2,000	USD 1,350
Smile Designing	USD 8,000	USD 1,100
Metal Free Bridge	USD 5,500	USD 600
Dental Implants	USD 3,500	USD 900
Porcelain Metal Bridge	USD 3,000	USD 600
Porcelain Metal Crown	USD 1,000	USD 100
Tooth Impactions	USD 2,000	USD 125
Root Canal Treatment	USD 1,000	USD 110
Tooth Whitening	USD 800	USD 125
Tooth Colored Composite	USD 500	USD 30
Fillings / Tooth Cleaning	USD 300	USD 90

The important question here is for whom is 'cost effective' services to be provided. Clearly the services are "cost effective" for those who can pay and in addition come from countries where medical care costs are exorbitant—because of the failure of the government to provide affordable medical care. It thus attracts only a small fraction that can pay for medical care and leaves out large sections that are denied medical care but cannot afford to pay. The demand for cost effective specialized care is coming from the developed countries where there has been a decline in public spending and rise in life expectancy and non-communicable diseases that requires specialist services.

Table 3. Medical Procedure Charges in India & USA

Procedure	*United Kingdom (USD) Approx*	*India (USD) Approx*
Open Heart Surgery	USD 18,000	USD 4,800
Cranio-Facial surgery and skull base	USD 13,000	USD 4,500
Neuro-surgery with Hypothermia	USD 21,000	USD 6,800
Complex spine surgery with implants	USD 13,000	USD 4,600
Simple Spine Surgery	USD 6,500	USD 2,300
Simple Brain Tumor -Biopsy -Surgery	USD 4,300 USD 10,000	USD 1,200 USD 4,600
Parkinsons - Lesion - DBS	USD 6,500 USD 26,000	USD 2,300 USD 17,800
Hip Replacement	USD 13,000	USD 4,500

Significant cost differences exist between U.K. and India when it comes to medical treatment. Accompanied with the cost are waiting times which exist in U.K. for patients which range from 3 months to over months. India is not only cheaper but the waiting time is almost nil. This is due to the outburst of the private sector which comprises of hospitals and clinics with the latest technology and best practitioners.

Markets tend to be bureaucratic and stifling when insurers or governments pay most medical bills. In the United States, third parties (insurers, employers and government) pay for about 87 percent of health care. So patients spend only 13 cents out of pocket for every dollar they spend on health care. As a result, they do not shop like consumers do when they are spending their own money, and the providers who serve them rarely compete for their business based on price.A much higher percentage of private health spending is out of pocket in countries with growing, entrepreneurial medical markets. For instance, patients pay 26 percent of health care spending out of pocket in Thailand, 51 percent in Mexico and 78 percent in India. When patients control more of their own health care spending, providers are more likely to compete for patients based on price. Consequently, these countries have more competitive private health care markets.

CII has also suggested that government should encourage medical tourism by increasing air connectivity linking major cities like Delhi, Chennai, Bangalore, Hyderabad and kolkata and create health support infrastructure. CII says that it is also essential to establish the Indian healthcare brand synonymous with safety, trust and excellence. There is a need to undertake an international marketing campaign targeted at select countries besides establishing one stop centers in key markets to facilitate the inflow of foreign patients. There is also a need to streamline immigration process for medical visitors.

The quality of healthcare for the poor in India is undeniably low. If India develops its infrastructure to international levels, it will be able to benefit medical services sector and more over help the world access the Indian medical services. The sight of the countries overcrowded public hospitals; open sewers and garbage littered streets would unsettle most visitors' confidence about public sanitation standards in India. Patients from the United States and Europe still are relatively rare not only because of the distance they must travel but also hospital executives acknowledge, because India continues to suffer from an image of poverty and poor hygiene that discourages many patients.

Table 4. Cost comparisons of different treatments in India with the developed countries.

Sl No	Treatment	Cost in the best hospitals of India	Cost in developed country
1	Complex heart operation	$8500 including airfare	$45000 in America
2	preventive health screening	$90	$600
3	Heart Surgery	$6500	$35000
4	Bone marrow transplant	$30000	$300000 in US
5	Open heart surgery	$15000	$200000 in US $75000 in Britain
6	Knee Surgery	$8000	$18500
7	Dental, Eye & Cosmetic Surgery	$y	$5y
8	Replacement of bulky heart valve	$12000	$300000
9	MRIS	$70	$850
10	Hip Resurfacing	$6000	$35000

Global competition is emerging in the health care industry. Wealthy patients from developing countries have long traveled to developed countries for high quality medical care. Now, a growing number of less-affluent patients from developed countries are traveling to regions once characterized as "third world." These patients are seeking high quality medical care at affordable prices. Reports on the number of patients traveling abroad for health care are scattered, but all tell the same story. An estimated 500,000 Americans traveled abroad for treatment in 2005. A majority traveled to Mexico and other Latin

American countries; but Americans were also among the estimated 250,000 foreign patients who sought care in Singapore, the 500,000 in India and as many as 1 million in Thailand. Global competition is emerging in the health care industry. Wealthy patients from developing countries have long traveled to developed countries for high quality medical care. Now, growing numbers of patients from developed countries are traveling for medical reasons to regions once characterized as "third world." Many of these "medical tourists" are not wealthy, but are seeking high quality medical care at affordable prices. To meet the demand, entrepreneurs are building technologically advanced facilities outside the United States, using foreign and domestic capital. They are hiring physicians, technicians and nurses trained to American and European standards, and where qualified personnel are not available locally, they are recruiting expatriates.

The medical industry on a commercial platform with tourism is a new and upcoming industry and needs to be explored. States like Karnataka, Kerala, Delhi, West Bengal and Maharastra are trying their best to woo foreign patients to India and to be amongst the most favourable health destination. There is a need for constant endeavor for other states to try their best to nurture themselves in this field and contribute to GDP by providing quality service.

Medical Tourism : Opportunities for India

World Tourism Indicators suggest that in 2002, number of International tourists reached the 700 million mark with arrivals to Asia and the Pacific 18.7%. Europe saw highest number of tourists. At that time, India did not figure in the top 10 international tourist destinations because India's share in Asia & Pacific region stands at a mere 1.8%

India is a recent entrant into medical tourism. As per research reports, approx. 150,000 medical tourists came to India in 2004 and according to a study by McKinsey and the Confederation of Indian Industry, medical tourism in India could become a $1 billion business by 2012. The report predicts that: "By 2012, if medical tourism were to reach 25 per cent of revenues of private up-market players, up to 2,297,794,117 USD will be added to the revenues of these players".

The Indian government predicts that India's $17-billion-a-year healthcare industry could grow 13 per cent in each of the next six years, boosted by medical tourism, which industry watchers say is growing at 30 per cent annually. This projection is largely based on the assumption that six hundred thousand Baby Boomers from the United States, Europe and Australia will age and seek medical care by that time.

Quality and Range of Services

India has number of hospitals offering world class treatments in nearly every medical sector such as cardiology and cardiothoracic surgery, joint replacement, orthopaedic surgery, gastroenterology, ophthalmology, transplants and urology to name a few. The various specialities covered are Neurology, Neurosurgery, Oncology, Ophthalmology, Rheumatology, Endocrinology, ENT, Paediatrics, Paediatric Surgery, Paediatric Neurology, Urology, Nephrology, Dermatology, Dentistry, Plastic Surgery, Gynaecology, Pulmonology, Psychiatry, General Medicine & General Surgery. For its quality of services and the infrastructure available, India is attracting a vast pool of tourists from the middle east, Africa etc.

As Indian corporate hospitals like Apollo, Max HealthCare, Fortis etc., are on par with the best hospitals in Thailand, Malaysia and Singapore there is scope for improvement, and the country is becoming a preferred medical destination

Manpower

India has a Large pool of doctors (approx. 600000), nurses & paramedics with required specialization and expertise and the language advantage (English speaking skills). The medical education system caters to the ever increasing demand for the delivery of the quality health care services all over the country.

The Price Advantage

For long promoted for its cultural and scenic beauty, India is now being put up on international map as a heaven for those seeking quality and affordable healthcare. With 50 million Americans without health insurance and the waiting lists for state-run facilities often endless in the UK, Canada and Europe, foreigners are increasingly flocking to India because it offers quality treatment at a fifth of the cost abroad.

In India, complicated surgical procedures are being done at 1/10th the cost as compare with the procedures in the developed countries. Not only this, the hospitals are well equipped to handle the data and information through computerized Hospital Information Systems. The hospitalization and the procedural price advantage also is supported by Lower Medication cost. If a liver transplant costs in the range of 137,867 USD - 160,845 USD in Europe and double that in the US, a few Indian hospitals have the wherewithal to do it in around 34,466 USD - 45,955 USD. Similarly, if a heart surgery in the US costs about Rs 45,955 USD, a leading Indian hospital will do it in roughly 4,595 USD.

Tourism Attraction

India has a 5000 year old civilization and is known for its cultural and religious diversity with Diverse geographical landmarks. The traditional arts and crafts add to its appeal as a tourists favourite. Along with this Indians enjoy freedom, vibrant democracy and women empowerment.

Alternative Therapy

India offers not just treatment but spiritual and mental healing as well. India needs to club together a couple of 'pathies' because it has a very strong base of alternative healing therapies like yoga, naturopathy, ayurveda Kerala's health retreats, etc.

No Waiting

In addition to the increasingly top class medical care, a big draw for foreign patients is also the very minimal or hardly any wait list as is common in European or American hospitals. Hospitals now are starting to attract foreign patients from industrialized countries, and especially from Britain, U.S.A, Canada, where patients are becoming fed up with long waits for elective surgery under overstretched government health plans.

Industrial Analysis

The Industry can be broadly classified into:

- *The Alternative Therapy Service*: which is available exclusively to India namely
    - Yoga
    - Naturopathy
    - Ayurveda
    - Yunani Medicine
    - Kerala Health Retreats
    - Meditation
- *The Corporate Health care Services*: provided by competent private hospitals like Apollo and Fortis

STATES PROMOTING HEALTH TOURISM

The Indian Ministry of Tourism has announced a number of incentives to give a fillip to the sector. It has identified 31 villages across the country to be developed as tourism hubs. The states in which these villages have been identified include Himachal Pradesh, Gujarat, Maharashtra, Bihar, Karnataka, Madhya Pradesh, Andhra Pradesh, Kerala, Tamil Nadu, Orissa, Assam, Sikkim, Rajasthan and West Bengal

Kerala

The Pioneer state Kerala, or God's Own Country as its corporate slogan goes, has pioneered health and medical tourism in India. They have made a concerted effort to promote health tourism in a big way, which has resulted in a substantial increase of visitor arrivals into the state. Kerala and Ayurveda have virtually become synonymous with each other. However, though Kerala has strongly focused on Ayurveda and its wide array of treatments and medications, good facilities are also available in the other traditional forms of medicine as well as in modern medical treatment. The bias towards health tourism in Kerala is so strong that Kerala Ayurveda Centres have been established at multiple locations in various metro cities, thus highlighting the advantages of Ayurveda in health management. The health tourism focus has seen Kerala participate in various trade shows and expos wherein the advantages of this traditional form of medicine are showcased. Kerala, India has one of the best qualified professionals in each and every field, Allopathi, Dental, Ayurveda, etc., and this fact has now been realized the world over. Regarding Medical facilities Kerala has the most competent doctors and world class medical facilities. With most competitive charges for treatment, Kerala is a very lucrative destination for people wanting to undergo treatment of certain medical problems who do not need immediate emergency treatment.

Kerala has established itself as a prominent Destination of world leisure tourism for its natural beauty and cultural assets. The growth of Tourism in Kerala has been induced by the buyer driven factors. The collective marketing effort through the tourism department has been limited. The scenario of Medical Tourism is also not much different from leisure tourism.Medical tourism in Kerala grew without much wilful collective effort. It was recognized as an opportunity by some sectors, particularly the Ayurveda sector who took some collective effort to convert Kerala as source for Ayurveda treatment. Then came Dentistry and Modern Medicine. A combination of many factors has led to the increase in popularity of medical tourism in Kerala:

— Traditional systems of medicine like Ayurveda and Siddha are widely popular in the state, and draws increasing numbers of tourists
— High costs of healthcare in industrialised nations
— Ease and affordability of international travel
— Improving technology and standards of care.

West Bengal

Kolkata, Aug 29: West Bengal, from where a large number of patients go to the southern states for specialised healthcare, is itself likely to become the hub of health hub of tourism in India soon. Three large super speciality hospitals with world-class facilities would come up in the state. West Bengal has produced many reputed doctors who are working in differents parts of the world and they have been invited to work at these hospitals.

Gujarat

Much of the NRI population, that is of Gujarati origin can take advantage of the medical facilities in Gujarat. Some of the major hospital groups such as Apollo already have a presence in Gujarat & others are looking for strategic cooperation include:

— *Sell side lead 1*: Is a leading institute, specializing in heart & orthodontics.

— *Sell side lead 2*: Is a leading dental institute, including cosmetic surgery.

— *Sell side lead 3*: Is a leading ophthalmology centre specializing in cataract surgery.

— *Sell side lead 4*: Is a leading multispeciality hospital.

Strategic View Point: Gujarat based healthcare providers are open to strategic alliances with hospitals, insurance & travel/ tour operators abroad that may refer patients from their countries of origin.. It is felt that many of the Gujarat based operators would have to align with national or international operators, possibly through a strategic stake to take full advantage of the medical tourism possibility.

Karnataka

Karnataka and especially Bangalore is now an acknowledged global medical destination. This is because of referral quality health services supported by qualified and experienced medical professionals, reputed medical research institutions, well connected for travel, conducive climate and cost of treatment being just one tenth that of global hospitals. Between 2005 end and 2006 August, the state has also witnessed a funding of 445 crore from leading corporate hospitals as a part of the brownfield and green field projects. These include a Rs. 200 crore from the Manipal Health Systems, Rs. 140 crore from Wockhardt Group of Hospitals, Rs. 100 crore from One World Hospital and Healing Centre promoted by Maureen Berlin and Rs. 5 crore by HealthCare Global Enterprises Limited (HCG), a leader in oncology care in the private sector in India.

Maharashtra

Maharashtra has a thriving tourism industry, and is now set to have a new kind of tourism -Medical Tourism. The FICCI Medical Tourism Council of Maharashtra is a dynamic initiative jointly undertaken by the Government of Maharashtra, the Federation of Indian Chambers of Commerce and Industry, the tourism industry and private as well as public health tourism providers.

FICCI Medical Tourism Council of Maharashtra has been founded with a clear mission in mind:

— To offer the world's best healthcare facilities coupled with the best heritage and tourist destinations.

— To show the world how to deliver "Value for Money" healthcare, with a human touch.

— To project Maharashtra as a synergysing destination for both medical academia as well as international medical conferences.

— To regulate and monitor the medical tourism sector and assist patients from abroad.

Maharashtra has all the necessary ingredients required to make medical tourism a success.

— A range of hospitals covering the entire spectrum of medical treatment.

— Over 70,000 highly qualified doctors, of whom 20,000 are specialists.

— 100,000 committed nurses and paramedical staff known for their care and compassion.

— Latest technology and equipment that supports a large number of medical investigations and treatments.

— Tourist spots that are supported by medical facilities, making them the ideal places for rest and recuperation.

CORPORATE HEALTH CARE SERVICE PROVIDERS

Medical tourism is predicted to double in the next few years as health services in India are a fraction of what they cost in the West. Apollo hospital gets 10-11 foreign patients every month. Five to seven per cent of Escorts' patients are from abroad. Though most of the traffic is from West Asia, southeast Asia and Africa, Indian corporate hospitals are networking with international health insurance companies so that these hospitals are recognised and Non Resident Indians can combine their treatment in India with family visits or tour to the country.

Apollo Hospitals Group

The Apollo Hospitals Group is today recognized as the "Architect of Healthcare" in India. Its history of accomplishments, with its unique ability of resource management and able deployment of technology and knowledge to the service of mankind, justifies its recognition in India and abroad. Their mission is "to bring healthcare of international standards within the reach of every individual. We are committed to the achievement and maintenance of excellence in education, research and healthcare for the benefit of humanity". Apollo's capabilities have received international acclaim resulting in the replication of its Indian models at international locations. Apollo group is also in talks with private healthcare groups and government authorities in Nigeria, South Africa, Tanzania, Mauritius, Yemen, Muscat, Bahrain, Vietnam, Malaysia, Thailand and other neighbouring countries to establish its presence.

Escorts Heart Institute & Research Centre

Escorts is steadily consolidating its presence in healthcare, which is likely to emerge as the largest service sector industry. Currently, Escorts is operating three large hospitals in New Delhi, Faridabad and Amritsar. Together with 11 heart command centres and associate hospitals, Escorts is managing nearly 900 beds. Escorts excellence in providing healthcare services has received due recognition. Escorts Heart Institute and Research Centre (EHIRC), New Delhi, has been ranked as the best cardiac hospital in India by an Outlook-Cfore survey and has been given the highest grade by CRISIL - an acknowledgement of the quality of delivered patient care.

EHIRC is a leader in the fields of cardiac surgery, interventional cardiology and cardiac diagnostics. The Institute has introduced innovative techniques of minimally invasive and robotic surgery. The

Institute's latest addition of state-of-the-art Cardiac Scan Centre providing a combined power of CV-MRI and Smart Score CT Scanner to diagnose coronary artery disease at its very early stage. This facility is the first of its kind outside America. State-of-the-art infrastructure and equipment has made this setup technically the largest and the best dedicated cardiac hospital in the world. The 332-bed Institute has nine operating rooms and carries out nearly 15,000 procedures every year.

Dr. Vivek Saggar's Dental Care & Cure Centre

Dental Care and Cure Centre is, centrally located in Ludhiana, easily approachable from any part of Punjab by rail or road. It takes not more then two hours from any part of Punjab to reach this place. Theirs is a 6 chair operatory with an in house dental lab, the Dental Caps, Crowns and Beyond Dental Lab, which has been designed on the European standards. The office has been designed to provide an environment of comfort that combines exceptional skill levels, a respectful approach to treatment, Clinical and technical excellence with an individualized care approach by providing the most advanced, optimal dental care to the best of our ability. Theirs is a full service cosmetic and general dental office specializing in creating beautiful smiles. The in house facility of Dental Caps, Crowns and Beyond... Dental Lab gives them the unmatched time advantage plus international quality control. For NRI's and foreigners they provide special care in the form of appointments at a short notice and the work is completed within the span of 3-5 days keeping in mind your tight schedule.

NM Excellence

NM Excellence was formed from one man's vision to provide a healthier future for the citizens of Mumbai. Established in 2001 by M.D. Radiologist Dr. Nilesh Shah, this modern and sophisticated preventive health checkup centre aims to revolutionize the way healthcare is perceived and practised in India. Backed by over two decades of diagnostic experience under the banner of NM Medical, NM Excellence employs the latest, top-of-the-line imagining modalities, operated by qualified and professional doctors, with a friendly and efficient staff to make a client's experience as memorable as possible. Having viewed the vast range of diseases that can be prevented if detected early enough through its diagnostic experience, NM Excellence philosophizes that a preventive health checkup in today's day and age is an absolute must. NM Excellence is one of Mumbai's foremost preventive healthcare centres boasting of top-of-the-line diagnostic equipment, highly qualified doctors, a well-trained service staff, and a professional yet warm environment that makes one feel at home immediately.

PD Hinduja National Hospital & Medical Research Centre

An ultramodern hospital on the busiest artery in Central Mumbai, PD Hinduja National Hospital & Medical Research Centre was established by the Hinduja Foundation in collaboration with Massachusetts General Hospital (MGH), Boston. The fulfilment of Founder Parmanand Deepchand Hinduja's dream, the 351-bed hospital offers comprehensive services covering the gamut from diagnosis and investigation to therapy, surgery and postoperative care. As a tertiary care hospital, the services offered are comprehensive covering investigation & diagnosis to therapy, surgery & postoperative care. The inpatient services are complemented with a day centre, outpatient facilities and an exclusive centre for health check for executives. Hinduja Hospital was the first multi disciplinary tertiary care hospital to have been awarded the prestigious ISO 9002 Certification from KEMA of Netherlands for Quality Management System

LV Prasad Eye Institute

Set up as a not-for-profit trust, LVPEI has now come a long way in its journey towards realizing these goals. However, our changing world continues to throw up new challenges and new threats to health, and LVPEI too continues to search for ways in which these challenges can be overcome, in the field of eye health. In partnership with international health organizations such as the World Health Organisation and the International Agency for the Prevention of Blindness, LVPEI designs and implements innovative eye health programmes that reach people in the most remote rural areas. While the range of our research and training activities is international, our focus is on bringing this quality of care to the poorest segments of India and the developing world. Our successes include the establishment of rural eye health centres that provide high-quality eye care at the lowest possible cost, or at no cost to those to whom such care would otherwise be inaccessible.

Cord Blood Banking Opportunities

Cord Blood –i.e. the blood that remains in the umbilical cord after a baby is born-represents a new and the richest source of stem cells-which is the origin of the body's immune & blood system. With rising interest in stem cell based therapy, the scope of cord blood bank is becoming more of a cell pharmacy. In order to understand the importance and potential of Cord Blood Banking, it is imperative to explore further the emerging applications of stem cells.

Stem cells are basically the primal cells found in the multi cellular organisms. It has the remarkable potential to develop into many different cell types in the body, serving as a sort of repair system for the body. They are actually master cells because they give rise to all tissues, organs and system in the body. The stem cells ability to differentiate or change into other types of cells in the body is a new discovery that holds tremendous potential for treating and curing some of the most common diseases such as heart diseases, cancer etc.

There are basically three sources of stem cells; *bone marrow, embryonic cells and cord blood.* A bone marrow based surgical treatment is mostly stringent and is a difficult process, as it requires accurate and correct match which is often too tedious. On the other hand the treatment based on embryonic cells involves a lot of controversies as it requires the culture of embryo or waste fetus. The third and the richest source of stem cells is the cord blood. According to Weiss et al, umbilical cord blood contains inexhaustible, noncontroversial sources of stem cells for therapy.

Stem cell therapy in the coming decades may provide solutions to incurable ailments and severe injuries. Diseases like leukemia, metabolic disorders and immune deficiencies etc have been successfully treated with umbilical cord blood transplantation. Further stem cell breakthrough is expected to promote effective low cost treatment for diseases like diabetes, stroke, spinal cord damage etc.

The Indian Council of Medical Research has estimated that some 50 million patients with heart disease, 5 million with Parkinson's disease and 5 million with Alzheimer's disease in India are 'potential beneficiaries' of stem cell therapy. First-generation therapy is already being offered in South Korea for spinal injuries. Some of the current and emerging applications of cord blood based stem cells have been listed in Table 5, below.

Table 5. Applications of Stem Cells

Current Applications of Stem Cells/Cord blood	*Emerging Stem Cell /Cord blood Applications*
Acute Leukemias	Cardiac Disease
Chronic Leukemias	Diabetes
Thalassemia	Multiple Sclerosis
Fanconi's Anemia	Muscular Dystrophy
Sickle Cell Anemia	Parkinson's Disease
Hodgkin's Lymphoma	Spinal Cord Injury
Non-Hodgkin's Lymphoma	Stroke
Multiple Myeloma	Alzheimer's Disease
Others	Lupus,Rheumatoid Arthritis

Cord blood is the blood that remains in the baby's umbilical cord after it has been cut and is a rich source of stem cells. Earlier treated as a waste to be discarded after birth, cord blood is now considered a precious resource. Although the first cord blood transplant was performed by Gluckman in 1988, the concept of banking cord blood was pioneered by Dr. Pablo Rubinstein, who was awarded grant by the National Institute of Health to set up the first National Cord Blood Banking Program at the New York Blood Centre.

Back home in India, umbilical cord research started in 1990 at Cancer Research Institute, Mumbai, but did not receive any support from the government to set up a stem cell bank. The first private stem cell bank in India, however, was set up in 2002.

A cord blood bank is place that stores umbilical cord blood for future use. Cord blood banking basically involves three steps: *collection, processing and storage*. Cord blood collection is a simple, safe and painless procedure that usually takes less than 5 minutes and can be performed just after child birth in which the cord is clamped and cut and the blood is drawn from the umbilical cord in a specialized bar coded bag. These collections are further harvested for stem cells, which are then stored in cryo-vials at -196 degrees celsius in liquid nitrogen

Cord blood banks can be primarily divided into public and private banks. While public banks accept eligible donations to be used for anyone in need; private banks allow families to preserve their blood for their own use for a fee ($800-$2000). The basic differences between a public and a private cord blood bank have been enumerated in Table 6.

Table 6. Types of Cord Blood Banks

Public banks	Private banks
i. Use not restricted.	i. For use of the family
ii. No remuneration collected.	ii. Facility paid for by the family.
iii. Usage subject to availability	iii. Availability guaranteed

The medical community strongly supports public cord blood banking as it widens the compass of beneficiaries from medical advances. However, since the estimated probability of a need for cord blood stem cells within a family is 1/1500, private cord blood banking is generally not recommended. Globally, out of 100 cord blood stem cell banks, 75 are public banks.

Major Players in Cord blood Banking

The major players of cord blood banking in India are *Relicord, Lifecell, and Histostem Histostem Co. Ltd*., is a South Korean, US based Biotechnology Company that is developing the latest human cell based therapy. It is a pioneer in cell based therapy. The main divisions of Histostem are cell therapy research, public cord blood bank for transplantation, and family cord blood bank. It is in the process of investing $20 million to establish the world's largest cord blood bank,providing stem cells for transplant surgeons globally.

The leading Indian player in cord blood banking and cell research is Chennai based *LifeCell*. Establish with initial investment of Rs.140 million, LifeCell has a lab and state of art storage facility near Chennai. The world class infrastructure, which has accreditation from American Association of Blood Banks, help LifeCell provide seamless service from the collection of cord blood to harvesting, testing and finally storage. With 20 regional centres LifeCell has been able to harvest 10,000 units of stem cells.

The third important player is *Relicord*- which is Reliance Life Sciences Stem Cell Banking services has established south Asia's first most advanced and completely automated stem cell enriched umbilical cord blood repository. This is the first cord blood repository in the world to be accorded a license by an official regulatory authority, Food and Drug Administration (FDA), Government of India.

In order to boost medical tourism, cord *blood banking* is geared to make a major contribution to the country with Histostem announcing to set up the world's largest cord blood bank in the country. Thus, after space technology and information technology, India is now all set to usher in new revolution in regenerative medicine.

Apollo Group of Hospitals in India a major player in the medical tourism arena signed a Memorandum of Understanding (MoU) with Histostem Inc, to offer stem cell therapy to patients from South Asia.. Histostem and Apollo together will establish and operate treatment centres known as Histostem Cell Treatment Centres. Apollo's doctors and nurses will be trained with the help of faculty from Histostem to provide stem cell therapy protocol and help develop new treatments. Histostem has also entered into an agreement with the state governments for setting up a National (Umbilical) Cord Bank in Mumbai, Delhi, Chennai and Kolkata.

High birth rate and lack of any stringent government regulations are the factors favouring the development of cord blood banking in India. With approximately 72000 births daily, resulting in discarding of 72000 umbilical cords a day-the storage of stem cell rich blood derived from these umbilical cords can prove to be the best possible insurance against life threatening diseases. The Ministry of Health has approved a Grant of Rs.5 crores to upgrade its stem cell research at the Mumbai based National Institute for Research in Reproductive Health under the Indian Council of Medical Research (ICMR).

New private cord blood banks are being established all over India in an attempt to use their knowledge, research and storage facility to benefit the Indian population. What seemed like a dream few years back is now becoming a reality. The use of umbilical stem cells for therapeutic purposes can ensure lower treatment costs and longer lives.

Potential Scenarios for Cord Blood Banking

The extent of cord blood banking triggering boom in medical tourism seems to depend on two basic uncertainties.

— Size of global surgical treatment market captured by India

— Rate of growth in Cord Blood Banking in India

The potential scenarios based on the above two key parameters are :

— *Preferred Scenario-2020: India —The Enabler—a Global Health Destination*: Realizing the potential in cord blood based treatment, India seized the opportunity with both hands. On one hand the health care majors strengthened their expertise in surgical treatments and could market it globally. On the other hand players in the cord blood banking arena, geared to capitalize on the emerging stem cell research, decided to increase their repositories of cord blood. Backed by high birth rate and favourable regulatory climate cord blood banks triggered the boom in medical tourism making India a global health destination

— *Positive Scenario-2020: India—The World's Supplier of Cord Blood*: Despite the competitive edge in surgical treatments, India could not market itself well in the global market due to lack of coordination among the syndicate service providers. Further due to increased competition from other countries and lack of adequate support from the government India could not attract greater number of medical tourists. The players in cord blood banking, however, realizing the potential of cord blood based treatment could build huge repositories as targeted further foreign players like Histostem, along with Indian players like Relicord and Lifecell, could leverage the opportunity making India the worlds' supplier of cord blood.

— *Pessimistic Scenario-2020: India—The Synergy Lost*: The competitive edge in surgical treatments of major health care players were adequately harnessed and marketed well by India Inc., thus increasing its global share of cord blood based treatment from 0.33% to 10%. However due to lack of adequate supply of cord blood a critical input for such surgical treatments India loses out a major share to the competitors. Had cord blood banking sector been established simultaneously India could have captured additional 10% of the global share.

— *Worst Scenario-2020: India—The Paradise Lost-pportunities Lost*: Despite identifying the up coming opportunity in cord blood banking in surgical treatments, the stake holders of the sector could not leverage it further. Governmental bodies like ICMR, DBT, DCGI, could neither invest nor lay down proper policy for growth of cord blood banking in India. As a result India could manage just a marginal growth in cord blood banking. Further health care majors could not market itself despite distinct competitive advantage and failed to attract medical refugees. Today India stands on the sideline watching it competitors reap the benefits of the boom in cord blood based surgical treatment.

Actions Recommended for the Preferred Scenario

Given the scenarios discussed above, actions maybe recommended for the following stakeholders to help emerge India as the "Global Health Destination" the preferred scenario.

— *Cord Blood Banks-like*: LifeCell, Reliance Life Sciences, Cryobank, Histostem, etc have already geared up to capitalize on the upcoming potential. The need of the hour is to increase the number of repository of cord blood samples. To achieve this the actions recommended may include the following:

  — Building awareness establishing collection centres

  — Providing training for the specialized & contamination free collection process

  — Tie -up with hospitals engaged in cord blood based treatment

  — Diversify into public cord blood banking

— *Healthcare Majors*: like Apollo, Escorts, Hindujas, Fortis, etc need to be pro-active in not only facilitating the collection of the cord blood but also help in clinical trials and establish state of art to conduct cord blood based surgical treatments. Some of the actions recommended for them to realize the preferred scenario may be enumerated as follows:

- Strengthen their expertise in surgical treatments
- Market their expertise globally to increase the number of medical refugees visiting India
- Tie-up with syndicate service providers (travel & tourism sector) offering attractive packages to the medical tourists
- Tie-up with cord blood banks to have convenient access to the critical input for treatment

— *Government Bodies*-Indian Council of Medical Research (ICMR), Department of Biotechnology, and Drug Controller General of India (DCGI) are the major regulatory bodies responsible for formulating policies in this area. Some of the major strategic actions required to be undertaken by them are as follows:

- Issue guidelines on Umbilical cord blood banking facilities
- Facilitate Stem Cell Research through public-private partnership
- Encourage public cord blood banking to extend affordable treatment for all
- Favourable regulations for travel & tourism sector

— *Stem Cell research organizations*: are poised to play a significant role, given the fast pace of stem cell research. Increased outlay for research, public -private partnership and tie-up with the hospitals for clinical trials would further pave the way for faster growth in this arena.

Challenges to the Industry

India is emerging as an attractive, affordable destination for healthcare But there are some challenges that the country has overcome to become a tourist destination with competent health care industry:

Infrastructural Facilities

Indian hospitals must create exclusive infrastructure for corporate medical tourism:

— Chartered flight services, attractive tourism packages could be part of infrastructure

— There's growing pressure on U.S. corporates to reduce expenditure on healthcare

Foreign Customer Concerns and Expectations

The biggest challenge that the Indian hospitals face is assuring the foreign patients that they will receive quality care with no hidden costs.

The industry experts need to develop the decision making models through a thorough study on the factors that motivate the patients to choose India as a health care solution spot.

The basic expectations that the industry feels are important to be concerned about are:

— Hygiene

— Staff (trained technically as well as in soft skills)

— Customisation

— Insurance Cover

— Stability

— Connectivity

— International standard certification

Image of India needs to be Enhanced

The only one quality that Indian health industry lacks in is Health standards and hygiene. Indian hospitals lack accreditation from the Joint Commission on Accreditation of Healthcare Organisations (JCAHO), suffer from a lack of standards in terms of quality and rates for healthcare procedures, have no gradation system and a far from perfect insurance sector. In addition, top Indian hospitals have high infection and mortality rates, and are unwilling to disclose data regarding these.

Market Accessibility

The next challenge for the Indian industry is to make the Indian market accessible by tourist travel agents and websites of Indian health tourism. The government can play a vital part as the same can bring in lots of foreign revenue. The major ways of promoting our health tourism could be:

- Tourist companies of India
- Doctors of India visiting foreign countries
- International websites on Indian tourism
- Globalisation of marketing activities by Indian travel agents
- Tying up with foreign travel agents for promotion
- Insurance companies abroad who target customers

Excess Glamourisation of Health Care

It has been seen that the doctors and key player hospitals in India emphasis more on glamorization of health care than its actual advantages or research uniqueness. We need to work more on our research in medical field to be competent enough to beat our international competitor. In other words services should be given more attention and importance than packaging.

State Intervention

As this is a product which needs international tie-ups and international marketing, the state should help in the same. It should help the companies, hospitals and states in promoting health tourism abroad so that we can tap a wider range of customers.

Competition

Countries that actively promote medical tourism include Cuba, Costa Rica, Hungary, India, Israel, Jordan, Lithuania, Malaysia and Thailand. Belgium, Poland and Singapore are now entering the field. South Africa specializes in medical safaris-visit the country for a safari, with a stopover for plastic surgery, a nose job and a chance to see lions and elephants. Thus India has enough competition from the international market.This will be one of our major threats in bringing up and developing the health tourism industry.

Insurance Backup

One good way of tapping the foreign customers is tying up with Insurance companies abroad who could provide a genuine database of target customers.They can benefit from us by our services. Thus this would become a way of mutual marketing tactics between the Indian health tourism industry and the foreign Insurance agencies.

Local Demand vs Global Demand

It can be seen in case of hospitals like Apollo and Escorts that the Local demand itself to be catered to is vast. We should remember that we should have the facilities enough to manage the foreign customers not neglecting the local markets. Thus it is a challenge for both the Alternate therapy industry and Corporate Health Care Service Providers to cater to this vast market efficiently without compromises in quality on either side.

Future of Indian Medical Tourism

Today, medical tourism has become a worldwide multibillion-dollar industry, estimated to be $40 billion by 2010. With 220 million Baby Boom generations from U.S, Canada, Europe, Australia, and New Zealand aging by 2015, there seems to be a guaranteed market for inexpensive, high quality medical care. Although, India is a recent entrant into the medical tourism arena, it is poised to emerge as a major global player. As per research reports, approx. 150,000 medical tourists came to India in 2005 and the numbers are expected to increase at the rate of 28% in the coming years. In fact a study estimates that India has the potential to attract 1 billion medical tourists a year. Further, as per the study by McKinsey and the Confederation of Indian Industry, medical tourism in India is expected to become a Rs.100 billion ($2.2b) business by 2012. The Indian government predicts that India's $17-billion-a-year healthcare industry could grow 13 per cent in each of the next six years, boosted by medical tourism, which industry watchers say is growing at 30 per cent annually.

With India's top rated education system churning out 20,000-30,000 doctors and nurses every year and with half a dozen world class medical corporations serving medical tourists, the above predictions does not seem to be a distant reality, provided the stakeholders initiate the right move in the right direction.

India has emerged as one of the prime countries in surgical treatment and a hot spot for medical tourism. This is possible because of the cost effective criteria with same level of expertise as provided by the west. Some of the major players that are promoting excellent surgical treatment and a key destination for medical tourism.

However despite the distinct edge Indian hospitals have in surgical treatments, its share in cord blood based transplants is a meagre 0.25%. That is, out of the 7000-8000 cord blood transplants worldwide since 1993, only 20 such transplants have done in India so far.

Medical tourism growing at the rate of 30% annually has distinct competitive edge in surgical treatments.Despite medical expertise India's global share in cord blood based surgical treatment is a meagre 0.25%. (20 out of 8000 cord blood transplants). Major break through in stem cell research promising low cost treatment is attracting foreign players in India. While advancement in stem cell therapy would provide solutions to incurable and severe injuries, an established cord blood banking sector in the country would widen the compass of beneficiaries by making these affordable for the masses.

REFERENCES

Bookman and Bookman. (2007). *Medical Tourism in Developing Countries* New York: Palgrave Macmillan.

Cetron , M. .De Micco, F.J. and Davies, O. (2005) *Hospitality 2010: The Future of Hospitality and Travel,* Forecasting International , USA

Dastur, A. (2005). Umblical cord blood banking, *Journal of Obstetrics and gynecology of India,* Vol. 55, no. 6.

Government, Private Sector Chart Medical Tourism Direction, Business World. Manila. (2007).

Hutchinson, B. (2005). *Medical Tourism growing worldwide,* UDaily./ University of Delawre.

Malathy Iyer. (2004). "India Out to Heal the World," Times of India, October 26.

Marcelo, R. (2003). India Fosters Growing 'Medical Tourism' Sector, *The Financial Times*, July.

Prasad, R. (2004) Cord Blood:Biological Insurance, SciTech- Online Edition of The Hindu .

Woodman, J. (2007). *Patients Beyond Borders-Everybody's Guide to Affordable World Class Medical Tourism;* Catanoba Publishing, USA.

Watt, P. and Davis,.G. (2003) *Scenario : An Explorers' Guide* , Shell International Ltd, London

Rajghatta, C. (2007). Medical Tourism: Idiomatical American Sicko can reach out to India, by Knight Ridder, *Tribune Business News*. Washington.

6

Medical Travel and Trade in South East Asia

Medical travel refers to the international phenomenon of individuals travelling, often great distances, to access healthcare services that are otherwise not available due to high costs, long waiting lists or limited healthcare capacity in the country of origin. Increased foreign travel, increased availability of information to consumers worldwide and joint ventures in the private sector providing health services have all contributed to an increased consumption of health care abroad.

Medical travel is often referred to as medical tourism. However, medical tourism refers specifically to the increasing tendency among people from developed countries to undertake medical travel in combination with visiting tourist attractions. Medical tourism is often seen as adding medical services to common tourism. On the other hand, medical travel is more about extending healthcare services across international borders and expanding choices for patients on where to access health care. Health services in medical tourism packages are often provided through cost-effective private medical care for patients needing surgical and other forms of specialized treatment. This process is being facilitated by the corporate sector involved in medical care in collaboration with the tourism industry - both private and public.

Although medical tourism in its present form is a relatively new concept, medical travel is several thousand years old. One of the first recorded instances of medical travel dates back thousands of years to when pilgrims from the Mediterranean region travelled to a small territory in the Saronic Gulf called Epidaurus to visit the sanctuary of the healing god, Asklepios. While tending to their health requirements they also relaxed in the waters, enjoyed the wines of the regions and travelled within the area.

Western Europe has a long tradition of medical travel, going back to the water cures of the spas, where the healing mineral waters purportedly offered miracle cures for all known diseases. In the United Kingdom, dating back to Roman times, patients visited the waters at a shrine in Bath, a practice that still continues today. Moreover, and wealthy Europeans increasingly travelled to spas both in and outside of Europe. Until this time, medical travel had been primarily driven by those having the means to undertake such travel. This changed in the late nineteenth century. Florence Nightingale became one of the first people to promote medical travel as a means to find more affordable treatment when she started directing patients from the spas in Switzerland to the significantly less expensive spas of Turkey. In addition, she extensively documented and studied various aspects of her returning patients to assess the success of their medical tours, and made adjustments to the arrangements for future patients based on what she had learned.

In more recent history, health care is an area in which individuals have been taking advantage of globalization. This has been the case since the late 1970s. Initially, medical travel primarily consisted of wealthy individuals from developing countries who travelled to industrialized countries, like the United States of America, the United Kingdom and other European countries, to get specialized medical treatment at internationally renowned healthcare centres. This first phase of modern medical travel was characterized by the emergence of a private sector that thrived by servicing a small percentage of the population with the ability to buy medical care at the high end of the private medical sector.

At the end of the 1980s and in the early 1990s, medical travel began its development into its present form when the Cuban Government starting promoting medical travel as well as medical tourism as an industry, targeting countries such as Argentina, Chile, Mexico and Venezuela as its main markets. In this way, Cuba was the first country to systematically make a wide range of affordable medical services available to international patients, while at the same time demonstrating that the medical tourism industry could turn a significant profit. It is estimated that during the period 1997-1999, export of health services earned Cuba upwards of US$ 30 million. Other countries in that region like Argentina, Bolivia, Brazil, Colombia and Costa Rica quickly followed, specializing in meeting the increasing demand for affordable cosmetic surgery.

In the last decade, the medical travel movement has accelerated sharply. The present phase of modern medical travel is characterized by an industry approach whereby uninsured and underinsured consumers from industrialized countries seek first-class quality at developing country prices, a trend commonly referred to as medical outsourcing.

At the same time, the medical travel industry is increasingly grounded in tourism. Although exact statistics are not available, it is generally estimated that the present global medical tourism market is estimated to be approximately US$ 40 billion with an annual growth rate of 20 per cent. The International Trade Commission in Geneva says that medical tourism could grow into a US$ 188 billion global business by 2013.

Medical travel, in particular in combination with tourism, is turning out to be an immense business opportunity for nations that are positioning themselves appropriately. In 2005, India, Malaysia, Singapore and Thailand attracted over 2.5 million medical travellers. Hong Kong, China, Lithuania and South Africa are now emerging as major healthcare destinations. Many other nations, including Croatia, Greece, the Philippines and the Republic of Korea are also in the process of making themselves attractive healthcare destinations. The most recent trend is the expansion of medical tourism from specialized treatment to include a broader form of "wellness tourism".

There are several reasons for the increase in medical travel. First of all, the demographics of the developed nations are causing a significant increase in demand for health care. In Japan, the United States of America, the United Kingdom and many other European nations, the proportion of the population older than 60 years, in relation to the total population, is increasing rapidly. Similar trends are being seen in many countries across the world. At the same time, life expectancy in most countries has also increased steadily over the years;

the combined result is significant strain on national healthcare systems.

The inability of many healthcare systems to deal with the increase in demand does, in many cases, lead to compromised levels of service and decreased access through long waiting lists and high costs. This drives many individuals to seek alternatives to domestic health care. Such alternatives can be found in the economically stratified global healthcare marketplace, which offers everything from cutting-edge surgical procedures such as organ transplants to cosmetic procedures and wellness packages at a wide range of prices. As is the case in many economic sectors, outsourcing to more affordable health service provision abroad is increasing. Private healthcare facilities in countries such as India, Malaysia, Philippines, Singapore and Thailand are utilizing the prevailing cost differentials, relative to countries such as Canada, the United Kingdom and the United States of America, to attract international customers who have the financial means to access medical care abroad.

International accreditation and name recognition linked to quality care provision are laying to rest many of the concerns individuals may have regarding professional competence, patient safety and quality in low-cost health care abroad. Combined with inexpensive air travel, low-cost telecommunications, digitized patient records, widespread access to information through the internet, and an increasingly sophisticated medical travel industry to manage all these processes on the patient's behalf, travelling abroad for medical treatment is an appealing alternative for uninsured or underinsured individuals.

The alternatives available through medical travel are not only within reach of individuals in developed countries but also to people from developing and least developed countries who have the financial means to find sophisticated and affordable medical care in neighbouring countries.

It is possible to categorize present-day medical travellers into 4 main groups. The first group includes patients from developed countries who do not have, or have inadequate, health insurance coverage. Many of these individuals come from Australia, Europe and Japan, with the majority coming from the United States of America.

For example, in 2003, the number of people without health insurance coverage in the United States of America was 45 million, which translates to 15.6 per cent of the total population, and in 2005 the number of individuals without dental coverage in the United States of America was estimated at 120 million.

The second group includes individuals, also primarily from developed countries such as Canada and the United Kingdom, who face long waiting lists for non-elective surgery and other critical procedures. In the United Kingdom, many individuals choose to pay for medical treatment abroad to avoid long waiting lists even though the national healthcare system, in spite of being overstretched, ensures free treatment to all its citizens.

The third group includes individuals looking for affordable cosmetic procedures. Many of these individuals come from Australia, Europe and Japan, with a significant number again coming from the United States of America. For example, most health insurance in the United States of America covers critical care, not cosmetic care and beauty treatments. The increased demand for surgical procedures such as face-lifts, hair transplants, dental treatment and liposuction, as well as nonsurgical procedures such as botox and hair removal, and the relatively high cost of these procedures is driving many individuals to find more affordable alternatives abroad.

The fourth and final group of medical travellers includes individuals seeking quality-assured, often specialized, care that is unavailable or in short supply in their own countries. A significant number comes from the Middle East. An agency in Saudi Arabia estimated that every year, more than 500,000 people from the Middle East travel seeking medical treatment for everything from open heart surgery to infertility treatment. Destinations range from neighbouring countries such as Bahrain, Jordan, and Saudi Arabia to more distant countries like India, Malaysia, Thailand and the United States of America.

This last group also includes an increasing number of medical travellers from developing and least developed countries seeking better healthcare infrastructure at affordable prices in their own neighbourhood. A significant majority of the medical travellers to Jordan come from neighbouring countries with poor medical infrastructure facilities. Many people from Bangladesh and Nepal go to India for medical treatment. Medical travel from Indonesia to Malaysia, Singapore and Thailand is also increasing. Of interesting note is the report of Nigerians spending an estimated US$ 1 billion a year on health care outside of their country. Whereas ten years ago, most of this money was spent in Europe and America, it is now increasingly directed to developing countries with advanced facilities at reasonable prices.

Medical Travel and Trade

Medical travel takes place within the overarching framework of international trade rules. The World health Organization (WHO) recognized the linkages with trade in the early 1990s following the success of Cuba. The WTO aims to reduce trade barriers, including in the field of health. The main WTO agreements related to health include the Agreements on Technical Barriers to Trade, the Agreement on Sanitary and Phytosanitary Measures, the Agreement on Trade-Related Intellectual Property Rights (TRIPS) and the General Agreement on Trade in Services (GATS).

Of 12 service sectors included in GATS, at least five are directly related to healthcare systems. The professional services under the business service sector deal with services of health professionals. The distribution service sector relates to services in pharmaceutical retailing. The education service sector involves the training and education of health professionals. The financial sector deals with health insurance and flows of foreign capital for investment in private hospitals. The health and social services sector includes hospital services, medical and dental services, diagnostic services and management of health service facilities.

Medical travel is covered under mode 2 of GATS. Mode 2 is one of the four modes related to trade in healthcare services worldwide. So far, medical travel is the most visible face of the increasing global trade in healthcare services, but the other three modes are expected to increase in significance in the coming years. There are various kinds of barriers to trade in health services. The main barrier is the non-portability of health insurance under mode 2. Others include entry visas, work permits, professional and premises licenses, investment permits and insurance reimbursement. Commitment to trade agreements for services can reduce some or all of these barriers.

A key element in GATS is that countries, although not obliged to do so, are encouraged to open sectors to trade. Although, a number of countries have already done so for health services, the impact of GATS in driving the privatization of health services has so far remained limited. However, this is expected to change. The WTO is increasing the sanctions for not offering to open sectors, by insisting that states must prove they are not using anti-competitive policies to protect a sector. This has the potential to contribute to the development of medical travel as there will be increased opportunities for investment abroad by healthcare service providers, but at the same time it poses significant challenges for national health systems.

The South-East Medical Travel Industry

Well-developed healthcare systems and advances in technology have supported medical travel among Western countries for many years. However, medical travel in Asia is relatively new, mostly emerging in the aftermath of the Asian financial crisis in 1997.

With the middle-class clientele in many countries affected by the economic downturn, private hospitals were faced with a significant drop in local business. Hospitals needed to be creative in identifying alternative sources of revenue. Their first steps into the international patient market were facilitated by their devalued currencies, providing an attractive combination of modern facilities and low prices. Thailand's Bumrungrad Hospital was among the first in the region to focus on attracting foreign patients, enticing hospitals in other countries to follow suit.

Although primarily driven by the private sector, including hospitals and intermediary organizations such as specialized travel agencies utilizing competitive marketing initiatives, governments are increasingly contributing to the development of this industry in South-East and East Asia. For example, the Malaysian Government has exerted its leadership to facilitate and encourage industry development, with the formation of the National Committee for the Promotion of Health Tourism. The Government of Hong Kong, China is starting to consider the possibility of marketing its traditional Chinese medicine capabilities to the region.

Singapore

Singapore is well known for performing complex neurosurgical procedures and delivering cutting-edge medical treatment by the region's leading health specialists, including surgeries such as liver and heart transplants. Its reputation for high-quality medical facilities and well-trained doctors pulled in more than 370,000 international patients in 2005. In 2006, over 410,000 patients from 60 countries came to Singapore for medical treatment. That same year, an additional 56,000 had medical treatment while already visiting the country.

Many patients come to Singapore from neighbouring countries, such as Indonesia and Malaysia. Patient numbers from China and the Middle East to Singapore are also seeing fast growth. Patients from developed countries such as the United States of America are increasingly choosing Singapore as their medical travel destination for its relatively affordable healthcare services and clean cosmopolitan image.

Singapore is Asia's leading medical hub, with advanced research capabilities as well as nine hospitals and two medical centres that have obtained JCI accreditation. It is also the oldest destination for modern medical travel in the region. The upper-middle classes from neighbouring countries like Indonesia and Malaysia have been utilizing Singapore's medical centres since the 1980s.

Singapore was not as badly affected during the 1997 Asian financial crisis as its neighbours; domestic financing for health care remained largely intact. However, due to the significant impact of the financial crisis on Singapore's major medical travel source countries, Indonesia and Malaysia, the number of foreign patients fell by more than a third between 1997 and 1998. As a result, Singapore was forced to tap into international markets farther from home.

Government support for medical travel in Singapore can be considered exceptionally strong. Singapore Medicine, a multi-agency government initiative, launched by the Acting Minister of Health on 20 October 2003, leads and coordinates the medical travel drive.

Singapore Medicine identified three key growth areas: heart, eye and cancer treatment. The initiative brings together the Economic Development Board, which promotes new investments in the healthcare industry, the Singapore Tourism Board, which is in charge of marketing, strengthening service delivery, and developing overseas referral channels, and the International Enterprise Singapore, which promotes the growth and expansion of Singapore's healthcare players.

Medical travel is perceived as a positive development in Singapore because its own population can benefit from the critical mass for specialization and sub-specialization, retention of medical and professional manpower as well as acquisition of new technology. Increased revenues and extension of benefits to the medical community are other benefits. Singapore sees medical travel as part of a larger economy/ecology.

In response to the increased competition from India, Malaysia and Thailand, Singapore has increased its efforts, with agreements signed at the governmental level with some Middle Eastern countries, including Bahrain and the United Arab Emirates in 2003. In January 2007, Singapore's Government announced that it would further step up its efforts to draw more foreign patients from outside South-East Asia to strengthen its role as a top provider of quality healthcare services in the region. Singapore's Health Minister even announced in parliament recently that Singapore would give priority to hospitals when it came to buying land. The Singapore Government plans to invest US$ 974 million in medical research and has hired McKinsey & Co. to consult on its Singapore Medicine project to increase progress towards its goal of attracting 1 million foreign patients by 2012.

Philippines

The Philippines has been quick to recognize the opportunities of medical travel. Given its high-quality medical labour force and competitive cost of service, the Philippines is working toward becoming the next hub for medical travel in Asia through the launch of the Philippine Medical Tourism Program (PMTP) in 2004. As of the end of 2005, the Program had received tourists from China, Japan and the Republic of Korea in Asia, and France, Germany and the Netherlands in Europe, as well as the United States of America.

The PMTP aims to strengthen the medical service market to increase its capacity to cater to international patients and to attract 700,000 medical travellers annually, to achieve almost PHP 1 billion in revenues. The Program is also seen as a key strategy to address the exodus of medical professionals from the Philippines by creating job opportunities for medical professionals at home.

Table 1. 2006 price comparison: The Philippines and the United States of America (US$)

Treatment	United States of America	Philippines
General medical checkup	5,000	500
Coronary bypass surgery	50,000	25,000
Kidney transplantation	150,000	25,000
Lasik eye surgery	3,000	1,000
Breast augmentation	5,000	2,000

The PMTP includes four key areas: medical and surgical care; traditional and alternative health care; health and wellness; and international retirement health zones. As part of the PMTP, the Department of Health has also included medical travel in the 2006 investments priorities plan and also introduced the concept of international medical zones. These zones are selected areas developed into centres of professional health care.

The PMTP is not only led by the Government, its current 27 partner hospital and clinics include government and private health facilities among its participants. Another key player in the PMTP is the National Kidney and Transplant Institute (NKTI), which attracts international patients from Australia, Canada, Israel, Micronesia, the United Kingdom, and several Middle-Eastern states. The NKTI, which is ISO 9001 accredited, is best known for its transplant programme for the kidney, liver, pancreas, stem cells and bone marrow. In 2006, the hospital's gross revenue increased by 22 per cent. In parallel to catering to international patients, the NKTI also provides free health care to domestic patients. In 2006, the provision of free services exceeded the annual government subsidy of PhP 185 million for free health care.

It is interesting to note that before 2005, NKTI had to use part of that subsidy to cover operational expenses. However, because of improved revenues, partly a result of its modest yet steady stream of foreign patients, the hospital was able to spend more on its indigent patients last year, and even put into the charity pot 20 centavos for every peso it received from the Government.

Thailand

Thailand was particularly hard hit by the financial crisis in 1997. To compensate for the significant drop in revenues caused by the economic crash, private hospitals started to explore the business of treating overseas patients. Since then certain private hospitals have had considerable success in tapping the international patient market with their affordable pricing of medical procedures.

The number of international patients visiting Thailand has increased from 500,000 patients in 2001; to 630,000 patients in 2002; 1,103,095 patients in 2004; and 1.25 million in 2005. In 2006, thirty private hospitals in Thailand accommodated 1.4 million international patients; this generated a total turnover of an estimated US$ 1 billion. The number of medical tourists is increased to 2 million in 2007.

The Thai Department of Export Promotion believes that the international accreditation of the Thai healthcare industry and the advanced medical technology, competent healthcare professionals and the reasonable cost for medical services are the main factors attributable to the increase in the number of foreign patients visiting Thailand. The international patients who visit Thailand for medical treatment are classified by the Thailand Department of Export Promotion, Ministry of Commerce, into three broad groups:

— *Expatriate:* comprising foreigners who work in Thailand and its neighbouring countries. These patients are generally treated for heart disease, blood-pressure, and respiratory conditions, as well as seeking plastic surgery;

— *Direct fly-in:* comprising foreigners who visit Thailand specifically to utilize the Thai healthcare services. These patients generally use healthcare services for heart disease, neurosurgery, eye care and kidney disease;

— *Tourist:* comprising foreigners who are tourists in Thailand and require Thai healthcare services for amongst other things, common diseases and respiratory care.

In June 2004, the Thai Government published its healthcare policy to develop and promote Thailand as the leading healthcare provider in Asia by the year 2010. The government strategy sought to increase marketing and public relations to foreigners, improve management, and develop healthcare products and services. The areas in Thailand which are being promoted as international healthcare centres are Bangkok, Chiang Mai, Koh Samui and Phuket.

The Thai Ministry of Public Health is working closely with the Thai Ministry of Tourism to promote medical travel in Thailand. Moreover, Thailand and Malaysia are in the process of exploring joint-promotion of medical travel to beat competition from other countries. However, government initiatives are exceeded by efforts being made by the private hospitals in Thailand to attract medical travellers. Bangkok's Bumrungrad Hospital is the leader in the field and considered to be one of the frontrunners in medical travel worldwide, though a number of other hospital groups are also providing strong competition. Hospitals in Thailand offer a host of facilities such as assistance in interpretation from more than 10 languages, and assured quality through JCI accreditation.

Malaysia

Private health care in Malaysia had been on the rise since the 1980s. The 1997 Asian financial crisis caused a drop in domestic patients visiting private hospitals. As businesses faced the reality of the economic downturn, health benefits for employees were cut or even removed completely. The Malaysian currency dropped rapidly and overall purchasing power, including for health care, decreased. Some households could no longer afford expensive private medical insurance and reverted to public health care. In addition, the currency exchange rates at the time of the crisis caused the prices of imported medical supplies and equipment to rise. As clientele was also dropping, hospitals were unable to raise prices to compensate for increased operating costs and profit margins were badly affected. Private hospitals in Malaysia were forced to search for alternatives abroad.

In developing the medical travel industry and medical tourism in Malaysia, much is owed to the concerted and synergistic efforts by the various parties involved in the nation's health tourism think tank – the National Committee for the Promotion of Health Tourism, formed in 1998. This high-powered committee is chaired by the Director General of Health and the core team comprises the Ministry of Health; Ministry of Culture, Arts and Tourism; Tourism Malaysia; Ministry of International Trade and Industry; Malaysian External Trade Development Corporation (MATRADE); Association of Private Hospitals of Malaysia; and the Malaysian Association of Tour and Travel Agents. The committee is supported by various other stakeholders both from the healthcare and travel industries.

The committee has a two-pronged objective: to further raise the standards of care and of caregivers, which in turn will put Malaysia on the map as one of the most desirable healthcare destinations. Five subcommittees were formed to address the following key issues: identifying source countries to promote medical travel, and drawing up tax incentives, fee packaging, accreditation guidelines and advertising guidelines.

Furthermore, the Government of Malaysia takes an important lead in the marketing of medical travel and tourism overseas through trade missions and other promotional activities. Road shows and marketing promotions have been organized and carried out by MATRADE and Tourism Malaysia, both of which are government bodies. In the period 2001-2002, MATRADE organized at least three specialized healthcare missions to promote medical travel and tourism in Indonesia, Myanmar, Viet Nam and countries in the Middle East. In 2005, the schedule of promotional activities included various places in Cambodia, China, Indonesia, Viet Nam and countries in the Middle East.

While Singapore and Thailand have several years head start, Malaysia's hospitals are beginning to catch up. The number of foreign tourists seeking treatment in Malaysia generated about US$ 27 million in 2004. In 2005, the foreign patient market was estimated to be worth about MYR 154 million (US$ 1 = approximately MYR 3.6) and medical travel was expected to generate at least MYR 2 billion a year in national earnings by 2010. A 2006 market analysis estimated that the majority of foreign patients receiving medical treatment in Malaysia were from: Indonesia (72 per cent), Singapore (10 per cent), Japan (5 per cent) and West Asia (2 per cent).

The significant price gap is Malaysia's main advantage. The Government is focusing on this advantage, in renewing its push for medical travel as part of a wider effort to reduce the country's over-reliance on manufacturing. To attract more foreigners to seek private medical care in Malaysia, a Health Travel Unit was established under the Ministry of Health to improve the quality of health services. In its further effort to promote medical travel and tourism, the Ministry of Health is cooperating with private hospitals, tour agencies and other relevant bodies to come out with packages to attract more travellers to Malaysia. Currently, there are 34 private hospitals involved in medical travel, targeting less-developed markets such as Bangladesh, Indonesia, and Viet Nam, as well as Middle Eastern countries. Common treatments are in cardiology, cardiothoracic surgery, radiotherapy and radiology.

Key Players in the Medical Travel Industry

Medical travel operators can be divided into two groups. First, there are medical centres such as hospitals and clinics. Medical centres that actively attract international patients are not involved only in the medical procedure itself, but are, in many cases, also responsible for all patient logistics from arrival to departure. Often the hospitals involvement already starts before arrival with the processing of the visa requirements and only ends after departure with patient follow up.

The second group consists of medical travel facilitators who function like agents and associated service providers. These are often smaller companies with just a few people on their payroll and most of them have spread their risk by dealing with hospitals and clinics in a number of different countries. Those medical travel agents which are dealing exclusively with hospitals of only one country or region are exposed to the same risks as the hospitals with which they work. These facilitators offer global healthcare options that will enable international patients, primarily from Europe and the United States of America, to access international health care at a fraction of the cost of domestic care. By selling a type of medical value travel, they focus particularly on the self-insured patient. Some companies charge clients a flat rate commission or a percentage of the total cost of care. Others do not directly charge customers, but are paid by the hospitals to which their clients travel for care.

The companies typically provide experienced nurse case managers to assist patients with pre- and post-travel medical issues. They also help provide resources for follow-up care upon the patient's return. Medical travel packages can include all costs associated with medical care, air and ground transportation, hotel accommodation, provision of a cell phone in the destination country for ease of communication, practical assistance from a local company representative at the healthcare facility, travel arrangements for a companion, stays in nearby resorts during the postoperative recovery period and side trips to tourist destinations.

Most medical travel facilitators are relatively new companies. Services include all hospital and travel arrangements, including medical intake by registered nurses and doctors. The approach typically includes a single lump sum payment per patient. There is no mark up on hospital fees, airfare, or any other expenses. These facilitators work with hospitals that are either JCI or ISO accredited or otherwise affiliated with recognized medical institutes such as Harvard and Johns Hopkins.

Other companies specialize in providing a complete service for accessing affordable international medical care, including managing the medical scheduling process, and arranging all travel, ticketing, and coordination with destination managers. This company states that it only works with medical providers that are JCI certified. Some other companies help uninsured and underinsured consumers obtain more affordable dental care, medical specialty care, surgery and diagnostic testing, including in India, Singapore and Thailand.

Some companies link uninsured and self-insured Americans to affordable and quality health care in India, by partnering with India's leading hospitals – Apollo, Escorts and Wockhardt – that provide easy access to care, at a fraction of the costs in the United States of America. The cost of the medical procedure quoted to patients is all-inclusive. It includes transportation, case management, the cost of the procedure itself, medicines, hospitalization and all costs associated with onsite follow-up care. The companies are able to provide tourism services as part of a complete package at extra cost, by entering into referral agreements with hospitals, and promoting the business of these hospitals in North America by identifying, qualifying and referring patients to the Indian facility.

DRIVING FORCES

Increased Costs

One on the main drivers is demographic change. By 2015, the health of the vast baby boom generation, including 220 million people in Australia, Canada, Europe, New Zealand and the United States of America alone, will begin its slow but inevitable decline. However, many developed countries with high standards of health care are already struggling to maintain their standards under the increased strain of an ageing and more demanding population. This could lead to increased consumer costs through rationing and queuing, as is now the case in Canada and the United Kingdom.

Limited Medical Insurance Coverage

As demand for health care increases, the cost of medical insurance also increases. This leads to an increasing number of people who are uninsured and underinsured, like those in the United States of America. Health insurance coverage in many countries often excludes dental care and caps other high-cost procedures. In addition, elective surgery, such as increasingly popular cosmetic procedures, is often not covered by insurance. The overall increase in cost of healthcare provision in many developed countries represents an expanding market for inexpensive, high-quality medical care.

Affordable and Quality Alternatives

In the Asian and Pacific region, countries like India, Malaysia, Philippines, Singapore and Thailand are increasingly able to meet the demand for quality-assured medical care through first-class facilities and highly trained medical specialists, including in tertiary hospital care. Many of these medical professionals have been trained at world class institutions abroad. These hospitals offer highly-qualified and board-certified physicians, top tier nursing staff and medical technicians, and highly personalized care. This translates into high success rates for complicated surgery procedures and high patient satisfaction rates.

Furthermore, medical care provision in these countries comes at a significantly lower cost. Basic costs, including wage levels and hospital operation costs, are much lower compared to the United Kingdom and the United States of America, thereby significantly reducing the costs of procedures.

Table 2. Indicative cost of surgical procedures (US$)

Procedure	United States	India	Thailand	Singapore
Gastric bypass	48,000	11,000	15,000	15,000
Heart bypass	122,000	10,000	12,000	20,000
Heart valve replacement	159,000	9,500	10,500	13,000
Hip replacement	44,000	9,000	12,000	12,000
Knee replacement	41,000	8,500	10,000	13,000
Mastectomy	24,000	7,500	9,000	12,400
Spinal fusion	63,000	5,500	7,000	9,000

Though costs vary considerably across countries and across institutions, a heart valve replacement that would cost US$ 160,000 in the United States of America may cost as little as US$ 10,000 in India, with airfare and a short vacation included. A metal free dental bridge costing US$ 5,500 would cost as little as US$ 500 in India or Thailand. A knee replacement can be performed in Thailand at one fifth the cost incurred in developed countries and Lasik eye surgery costing US$ 3,700 in the United States of America is available in many countries in Asia for around US$ 730.

Accreditation and Assurance

The standards of medical facilities all over the world are becoming increasingly transparent to the consumer through internationally recognized accreditation and certification schemes, such as JCI and ISO, as well as through international partnerships. Partnerships and managerial oversight from world-renowned medical providers like the Mayo and Cleveland Clinics, and Harvard Medical School, and partnerships with globally recognized insurance carriers contribute significantly to consumer trust. To gain consumer and industry facilitator confidence, and compete in the global healthcare market, medical institutions are increasingly seeking such accreditation and partnership.

Access to Information and ICT

The media buzz surrounding medical travel combined with the greater availability of information and use of ICT also significantly contributes to the increase in medical travel. The internet has played a key role in increasing access to information on services and costs worldwide. A wide range of websites are available that facilitate a variety of services ranging from selection of hospitals to making travel arrangements and booking all-inclusive medical travel packages. Through the internet, patients in other countries are able to learn about the many available options, compare costs and can easily contact providers in developing countries for detailed information.

The ability to research hospital accreditation and doctor's credentials, to review patient testimonials and communicate directly with service providers and medical specialists has further contributed to the ability of individuals to make informed choices. Email communication and electronic processing of bookings has also significantly reduced the run up time for a medical procedure abroad. In one example from Thailand, it is even possible to apply for visa extensions via a teleconference system, instead of going to the Immigration Bureau.

Telemedicine is an ICT application that has facilitated medical travel - enabling patient pre-screening and follow-up consultations for medical tourists. The Apollo and Wockhardt hospital groups in India are leaders in the field of telemedicine, using the technology both domestically and for international patients. This significantly increases the access to care, including for some of the most underserved populations like patients in closed prison settings. The electronic delivery of health services is expected to increase simply because it allows the provision of services without investing very heavily in infrastructure.

Niche Medical Services

The provision of niche medical services is another important driver of medical travel. International patients in need of specialized treatment are more likely to visit a destination that is well known for that specialty. Countries such as Singapore, which cannot compete on costs alone, position themselves as providers of high-quality care such as heart surgery and eye procedures, to wealthy patients from Asian countries who would have otherwise headed to reputable medical institutions in countries like the United States of America. Some hospitals in Singapore also focus on complex cases such as separation of conjoined twins in order to give them an edge and a sound reputation. Thailand has established a niche for itself for cosmetic surgery and dental procedures. The Philippines is best known for its renal care and transplants, with patients travelling from all over the world for kidney transplants.

Geopolitical Events

Wider political issues can influence where medical travellers will choose to seek out health care. For example, in recent years, medical travel to the United States of America has seen a significant shift to destinations in Asia.Prior to the incidents of 11 September 2001, the United States of America was a preferred destination for many patients from Middle Eastern countries. However, the difficulty in obtaining visas after that date has meant that a large part of this business has been diverted to other countries. Jordan has quickly positioned itself to receive much of the Middle Eastern patient load.

The number of patients from the Middle East to Hong Kong, China, India, Malaysia, Singapore and Thailand and has also increased. Easily available halal food and conveniences for practicing Muslims makes Malaysia a particularly attractive destination for Muslims, including those from the Middle East.

Industry Linkages

Increased cooperation between the different actors in medical travel is leading to greater flows of international patients. Hospitals are increasingly working with medical travel facilitators and traditional travel agencies to tap the international patient market, and link patients with competitive air fares and affordable vacation packages in exotic destinations. Such partnerships allow all players to focus on their core business, which, in the end, benefits the patient as well as the business interests of those involved.

Opportunities for Health Systems

Economic Gain

Medical travel contributes to the growth of health economies. It is a major source for foreign exchange and stimulates economic growth in other sectors as well, including tourism, transport, pharmaceuticals, hotels, food suppliers to hospitals and restaurants. The tourism market is particularly lucrative, as tourism is an integral part of service industries in many economies and an important source of foreign exchange. The labour-intensive nature of the tourism industry makes it an excellent generator of employment.

Reducing External Brain Drain

The international service trade has greatly affected the healthcare systems in developing countries. The last four decades were characterized by massive emigration of physicians from developing countries, such as Thailand and India, to developed countries, such as the United States of America, in response to increasing demand and higher wages. In this way, Thailand lost about 1,500 physicians, 20 per cent of its total number, in the period 1965-1975.

Anecdotal evidence from countries such as India and Thailand now indicates that large numbers of medical graduates, who acquired specialized medical degrees in developed countries, are finding it lucrative and more satisfying to return to their own countries.

Modern hospitals that make significant investment in facilities and staff, in part to compete for international patients, now also provide the benefits and working conditions to satisfy the aspirations of medical professionals who would otherwise move outside the country.

A good example is Bumrumgrad Hospital in Thailand; the majority of its 600 Thai health professionals has overseas training and certification, mainly in the United States of America, but preferred to return to work in Thailand. In India, increasing numbers of medical graduates trained abroad are also returning to practise in modern hospitals serving as medical tourism centres. It should be noted that Thai medical professionals are still travelling abroad for work. Except this time they are often travelling on behalf of their Thai employer to take up residency at the joint ventures medical centres that Thai private hospitals are increasingly investing in.

Improved Medical Infrastructure

Medical travel and the competition on the global health market promote technological advances and improved medical infrastructure. To attract international patients, hospitals must invest in high-quality facilities, cutting-edge technology and human resources. This necessity sets a higher standard for health care than many public hospitals are now measured against, and could drive public hospitals to invest in their own medical infrastructure and possibly revitalize weak healthcare systems.

International accreditation is sought by healthcare providers involved in medical travel, as well as demanded by patients and medical travel facilitators. In a number of countries, this has lead to increased emphasis on consistent good quality that may create pressure on other private healthcare providers and public facilities to emulate them, at least in part.

The medical travel centres in developing countries not only provide options for patients from developed countries, but also for medical professionals and patients from within the country and from neighbouring countries. Such centres provide stimulus for professional development, training and professional tenure within reach of the domestic population in terms of physical accessibility, and lesser costs compared to similar treatment in developed countries.

Challenges for Health Systems

Technocentric Approach to Health Care

Some researchers fear that medical travel would lead to what is known as a technocentric approach to health care. This is seen as a western concept, and something which would increase cost of healthcare delivery to the general public.

A generic problem with medical travel is that it reinforces the medicalised view of health care. By promoting the notion that medical services can be bought off the shelf from the lowest priced provider anywhere in the globe, it is perceived to take away the pressure from Governments to provide comprehensive health care to all of their citizens. The matter is further complicated by the competitive pressures brought on by private hospitals on the resource stricken public health systems. Investments in upgrading public health systems to keep up with the competitive pressures can translate into higher costs and thus limited accessibility for the general public.The development of traditional medicine systems through the promotion of holistic health packages to international patients have the potential to balance out the increasing technocratic approach to medicine in many developing countries.

Internal Brain Drain

An increase in the number of private hospitals, due to rapid economic growth or an investment in medical travel, can create an increase in demand for more doctors, which in turn can lead to internal brain drain from public health systems to private hospitals. As private hospitals expand to absorb the increasing number of medical travellers, they will need more medical and other professionals. In many cases, the top specialists in corporate hospitals are senior doctors drawn from the public sector. This has been observed in many countries where private and public hospitals coexist. For example, in Thailand, during the period 1988-1993, 21 rural district hospitals had to function without a single full-time physician due to internal brain drain. This trend was reversed immediately after the 1997 Asian financial crisis, when many doctors who had left the public sector returned to public hospitals because private hospitals had lost their middle class clientele. Presently, this trend has once again reversed.

Another important trend is the urbanization of health care. As part of the brain drain, more and more health professionals are being drawn to large urban centres, and within them, to the large corporate-run specialty institutions. The urban concentration of health care providers is a well-known fact; 59 per cent of India's practitioners (73 per cent being allopathic) are located in cities, and especially metropolitan ones. In Thailand, in 2006, around 35 per cent of the country's medical doctors were based in Bangkok.

Regulatory System

Medical procedures performed under medical travel carry some risks that local procedures do not. With surgery conducted as part of medical travel, a follow-up may be a problem and complications, side effects and postoperative care become the responsibility of the patient's home country. Should serious complications arise, patients might not be covered by insurance due to lack of insurance portability or might not be able to seek compensation via malpractice lawsuits. New insurance products that protect the patient in the event of medical malpractice occurring overseas are available but with higher cost implications.

Some of the destination countries do not have strong malpractice laws, so the patient has little recourse to local courts or medical boards in case surgery or a procedure go wrong. Other medical travel destinations do provide some form of legal remedies for medical malpractice. However, this legal avenue is often unappealing to the medical traveller who plans to spend only a short time in the country. Advocates of medical travel advise prospective travellers to evaluate the unlikely legal challenges against the benefits of such a trip before undergoing any surgery abroad.

Quality issues also continue to be raised in regard to local regulation covering medical treatment, including facility management and human resources. While many hospitals indicate that their specialists have been trained in Western nations, there is less assurance that training is maintained according to current standards and that nursing and other staff are equally qualified. The importance of this issue may loose its significance as more and more accreditations are given to the medical service providers by renowned agencies, organizations and institutes.

Health Equity and Ethics

There are increasing ethical issues with greater degrees of medical travel. The prioritisation of international patients over domestic patients when public health care is often not able to support the needs of domestic patients has raised serious concerns. Some critics point to the creation of a two-tier system for healthcare delivery that increases inequalities in healthcare access between private and public systems; sophisticated hospitals with the latest technology cater to the rich and the foreign tourists, while underfunded public health systems are left to cater to the poor who cannot afford access to these new hospitals.

Related to the issue of the stratification of healthcare systems, there exists the fear that subsidies to motivate private sector hospitals to get involved in medical travel will increase at the cost of spending on public health. In some countries in the region, the corporate private sector has already received considerable subsidies in the form of land purchase and reduced import duties for medical equipment. Some critics fear that the medical travel boom will only further legitimize their demands and put pressure on the Government to subsidize them even more.

The already scarce resources available for health then go into subsidizing the corporate sector. This can have serious consequences for health equity and the cost of services, and raises a very fundamental question: should developing countries subsidize the health care of developed countries? For example, in countries where both private and public hospitals are involved in government-promoted medical travel, critics fear that in light of expected revenue increases hospitals, both public and private, are shifting their attention, and most of their beds, to foreign patients. This highlights the need to consider implications of medical travel on public health systems and how the issues facing these entities could be effectively addressed to ensure comprehensive contributions from health systems to development.

Another example relates to organ transplants. Critics feel that programmes that encourage foreigners to have transplant operations may not only mean that local residents who need the same organs could be pushed down the waiting list; some of them say it could also lead to an organ-selling spree among the desperately poor.

On a broader ethical issue, even if the care is excellent, the question should sometimes be posed whether the procedures are actually medically necessary or are only undertaken to boost revenue. Pressure to maximize profits, in a competitive market where it is necessary to keep costs low, could have a dangerous effect on the quality of care and the image of the service provider.

Dependence on Foreign Clients

It is important to maintain a balanced portfolio of domestic and international patients to avoid the excessive reliance on revenue from international patients. Such revenue is less stable than that generated from domestic patients. Hospitals with mainly local patients face a lower business risk since their local clientele needs their services in uncertain times as well as in good times. While the income from elective procedures might shrink in a period of economic hardship, hospital survival is less likely threatened than that of a hospital which depends heavily on unpredictable foreign tourists and conducive environments for travel. However, the diversification in the composition of the clientele that includes patients from many different countries could compensate in, to some degree, minimizing the risk associated with dependency.

Domestic political changes and unrest, natural disasters like a tsunami or an earthquake, possible alterations of economic policies due to a change in leadership, as well as epidemics, such as SARS and avian influenza, can potentially affect the number of medical travellers and investors. Servicing bank loans and other financial commitments can become very difficult indeed if patients suddenly do not want to visit a country any more.

Despite this, many big hospitals and hospital groups aim to grow at up to 30 per cent per year and this is only possible if they further increase their share of foreign patients. The local market is just not growing fast enough to enable such medical institutions to maintain a balanced portfolio, and the hospitals have little choice but to increase their intake of international patients. However, as the dependency grows, so does the risk, especially in the current competitive market with many suitable alternatives for medical travellers. Many hospital groups have expanded into other less-familiar parts of Asia due to intense regional competition for foreign patients. On the other hand, such a situation can be one of the drivers in inducing Mode 3: Commercial Presence as the means to international trade in health services and facilitate regional expansion.

Regional Expansion

The medical travel industry in the ESCAP region is primarily centred on India, Malaysia, the Philippines, Singapore and Thailand, but is increasingly expanding to other parts of the region. Stakeholders in these countries are establishing linkages with the healthcare systems in other ESCAP member countries as well as in other regions, in particular the Middle East.

As these networks of healthcare providers expand, they create an international market of healthcare services. The synergy created by corporations expanding and integrating across national borders, in turn, encourages the further expansion of the medical travel market. One of the important reasons for healthcare corporations to acquire facilities in different countries is to use these facilities to refer and cross-refer patients: a hospital in Indonesia or Viet Nam may refer patients to another hospital in Singapore, where both hospitals are owned by the same corporate entity.

Given these developments, it is possible to look to other more advanced forms of regional integration to glean some lessons. The mobility of patients within the European Union is quite significant and the steps taken to manage them may provide valuable lessons to countries in the Asian and Pacific region, as they promote medical travel and protect access to health services to their own citizens.

Future Concerns

Medical travel is a comparatively recent phenomenon which is being seen in a group of countries which vary widely in economic development, but also in terms of development of their health systems. It is difficult to draw firm conclusions on the benefits and drawbacks of medical travel in different countries not only because of their widely differing socioeconomic situation, but also because of the absence of sound data and analysis. Therefore, the following recommendations are to be taken in the context of factors mentioned above.

Managing the Impact on Public Health Systems

— In some countries with low public expenditure on health, promotion of medical travel through indirect subsidies and tax exemptions has been criticized. Therefore, it should be ensured that (public) investments in medical travel benefit the public health system through mitigating policies which ensure a 'trickle down' effect and limit the cost to the public health system.

— Medical travel has been seen as contributing to an internal brain drain of professionals from the public to the private sector, though it has also been perceived as contributing to limiting the outward migration of health professionals by providing employment within the country. Therefore, policies for managing the mobility of medical professionals, both internal and external, are essential. These could be implemented through training and monetary incentives, as well as nonmonetary incentives, such as career development, Research and Development, specialization and medical professionals from the public sector working part time in the private sector.

— There is a need to strengthen ethics and professionalism among medical practitioners and other stakeholders in order to promote transparency and clarity in medical practice and management of information. This could be done through training on ethics and creating effective mechanisms for enforcement and through ensuring that health care is not driven by profit motives alone. Regional cooperation through country-level agreements on a common code of ethics could also be useful.

— Sentinel events, that may occur as an effect of medical travel in the receiving countries, need to be observed; these include:

  — Escalating costs in the healthcare system;

  — Irrational use of diagnostic technologies and techno-centric approaches to health care which may also contribute to the escalation of costs;

— Low staffing in public sector health care due to migration to the private sector, which services medical travellers.

Managing the Process of Medical Travel

— Medical travel is ongoing and the development of a national level evidence-based policy on it within the overall framework of health system performance, human resource availability, and ethical recruitment and health policy objectives is essential for it to be managed for the benefit of all concerned.

— Capacity building in the health sector, including on trade issues, would enable effective and informed participation of the health sector in crucial trade policy negotiations, and commitments on health-related issues could be made taking into account a public health perspective.

— Balanced policies and regulations can be used in order to manage patient flows in a manner that is beneficial to sending and receiving countries. Examples of enabling policies which have been implemented by countries in the region include liberalizing visa requirements for medical travel, tax benefits for development of the industry and agreements to allow greater mobility of professionals. Memorandums of Understanding between sending and receiving countries have also been useful in regulating flows and ensuring delivery of good quality treatment.

— Mutual recognition agreements for medical professionals at the inter-country level, including through national and international accreditation systems, could also play a role in smoother movement of professionals which would ensure that good quality of care is maintained.

— Implementation of policies and practices on consumer protection is also essential in order to manage the process of medical travel, especially with a focus on cross-border compensation and liability issues, and issues related to portability of health insurance. Measures to protect consumers could be encapsulated in an "International Patients Bill of Rights" as is currently under discussion in certain forums.

Regional Cooperation

Regional cooperation will mitigate the negative impact and will help to manage the process of medical travel. These include:

— Inter-country agreements on data collection and collation frameworks to enable cross country comparisons;

— Regional cooperation through country-level agreements on a common code of ethics for medical professionals and providers;

— Memorandums of Understanding between sending and receiving countries to regulate flows and ensure delivery of good quality treatment;

— Mutual recognition agreements for medical professionals at the inter-country level, including through national and international accreditation systems, to contribute to the smoother movement of professionals;

— Implementation of policies and practices on consumer protection as an essential way of managing the process of medical travel.

Medical travel, which refers to the international phenomenon of individuals travelling, often great distances, to access healthcare services that are otherwise not available due to high costs, long waiting lists or limited healthcare capacity in the country of origin, has been increasing in the Asian and Pacific region. Increased ease in travelling abroad, availability of information to consumers worldwide and joint ventures in the private sector providing health services have all contributed to increased consumption of health care abroad.

References

Avigail M. Olarte, (2006). "Health and the Philippines: And now hospitals as tourist spots", *Philippines Center for Investigative Journalism*, 12 September.

David Diaz Benavides, (2002). "Trade policies and export of health services: a development perspective" in Vieira Cesar ed., *Trade in Health Services: Global, Regional and Country Perspectives*. Washington D.C., PAHO.

Gupta Sen Amit, (2004). "Medical Tourism and Public Health", *People's Democracy,* 9 May, Vol. XXVIII No. 19

Philip Stevens, (2005)*Free trade for better health* (London, International Policy Network, accessed from <http://www.fnfasia.org/efn/publications/Trade&health_web.pdf

Prosenjit Datta and Gina S. Krishnan, (2003). "The Health Travellers", *BusinessWorld*, 22 December, accessed from <http://www.businessworldindia.com/issue/pharma.asp>.

Ray Marcelo, (2003). "India Fosters Growing 'Medical Tourism' Sector", *The Financial Times*, 2 July, accessed from <http://yaleglobal.yale.edu/display.article?id=2016>

Suwit Wibulpolprasert et al, (2004). "International service trade and its implications for human resources for health: a case study of Thailand", *Human Resources for Health*, Vol. 2, No. 10

Wee Sui Lee, (2007). "Medical tourism boosts Asian hospital shares", *The Bangkok Post*, 23 June.

7

Trade in Health Services: New Directions

Although there is significant investment for health care, the World Health Organization (WHO) recently reports that improvements in health status, coverage and access to care are not equally distributed between and within countries. Currently, the OECD countries spend US$3,000 billion annually on health, which is nearly 90% of total world health expenditure. Health care spending accounted for at least 8% of GDP in OECD countries, rising to 14% of GDP in the United States.

The annual per capita health care expenditure varies widely from US$3,500 in the U.S. and Switzerland to less than $5 per capita in sub-Saharan African countries. In the Caribbean, per capita health spending is $239 on average, from $44 per capita in Guyana, to $518 per person in the Bahamas. Health spending has generally been on the rise in the region: recurrent health spending increased from 4.2% to 5.8% of GDP in Barbados between 1994 and 1995.

Yet, the amount of health spending is not directly correlated with health status, as more health investment does not necessarily mean better health outcomes. For instance, while the U.S. has the highest investment in health among the OECD countries, the country ranks 37 in the world in terms of overall performance of the health sector. Countries such as Sri Lanka and Costa Rica appear to have higher returns to health investments than other developing countries.

On the demand side, the rising trend in real spending on health care is related to increases in life expectancy and the aging of the world population, resulting in longer periods required for medical attention.

In addition, there has been an increased prevalence of chronic conditions, such as diabetes and hypertension, which are costly to treat. Diseases, such as HIV/AIDS, have a significant impact on health care costs. Ministries of health face a dual challenge of caring for patients with chronic diseases, as well as controlling communicable and vector-borne diseases. This task places a financial strain on public health systems.

On the supply side, rising health care expenditures can be attributed to the introduction and indiscriminate use of expensive technologies; insufficient health care planning and coordination; and, lack of incentives to relate the cost of treatment to the expected health benefits. One of the major drivers for rising health care costs is the use of insurance to finance health care. Health insurance effectively separates the patient and the provider from the payment for services, so that there is little incentive to economize on both the use of services, and the intensity of care provided. Patients have a tendency to over-consume care, and providers have a tendency to prescribe a higher volume of diagnostic tests and ineffective procedures. Variable practice patterns by physicians can lead to wastage of health care spending on ineffective or inappropriate treatment by up to 60%.

The fiscal constraints faced by governments have led to health sector reform policies and programs, as well as identification with new sources of health care financing. Reform strategies have included organizational restructuring, decentralization, and improved management and administration of the public health care system, as well as concerted resource allocation toward more cost-effective and efficient health care services. The role of government as the primary provider of health care services is changing to one in which there is greater delegation of service delivery to the private sector. Government's role is now focusing more on policy formulation, regulation, and monitoring.

In the search for alternative sources of health care financing, the increased role of the private sector has become tantamount. In many developing countries, the private sector accounts for a growing share of health care spending. For instance, in the Caribbean, private health care spending is approximately 42% of total health care spending, ranging from 55% in Trinidad and Tobago to 25% in Suriname. (Table 1).

Table 1. Selected Indicators of Health Care Financing in the Caribbean

Country	GDP Capita (US$ 1995)	National Health Expenditure as a % of GDP	Per Capita National Health Expenditure	Share of Private Financing
Anguilla	$6,584	5.1%	$336	47%
Antigua & Barbuda	$8,110	6.1%	$496	39%
Bahamas	$11,940	4.3%	$518	42%
Barbados	$6,560	6.4%	$421	38%
Belize	$2,696	3.9%	$106	54%
Dominica	$2,990	6.6%	$198	40%
Grenada	$2,980	5.0%	$150	47%
Guyana	$590	7.5%	$44	31%
Jamaica	$1,510	5.0%	$76	51%
Montserrat	$5,893	6.5%	$383	37%
St. Kitts & Nevis	$5,170	5.6%	$289	43%
St. Lucia	$3,370	5.0%	$167	48%
St. Vincent & the Grenadines	$2,280	5.5%	$125	36%
Suriname	$1,118	8.0%	$95	25%
Trinidad & Tobago	$3,370	4.7%	$176	55%
Average	$4,344	5.7%	$239	42%
Range	$590 -$11,940	3.9% - 8.0%	$44 - $518	25% - 55%

In this era of globalization, another potential source of health financing is through the trade of health services on the international market. While trade in health services is not a recent phenomenon, it is becoming an area of greater strategic importance. For some countries, such as Cuba, Costa Rica, and Singapore, trade in health services is part of an integrated economic development and political strategy. Nevertheless, empirical evidence suggests that the volume of international trade in medical and health services is still relatively modest.

Benefits of Trade in Health Services

While health and social services have long been perceived as non-tradeable services to be provided by the public sector, there has been a change in this policy perception in some countries. There are several benefits to trade in health services. First, it is one means of earning much-needed foreign exchange. Revenues from the sale of health and health-related services can be used to:

— reduce the trade deficit in developing countries;

— purchase pharmaceuticals and supplies; and,

— import technologies into the health sector.

In theory, resources earned from trade in health services can reduce pressure on public sector financial resources, by either supplementing existing resources, or by substituting public for private resources in health care. Since much of the innovation related to trade in health services depends on private sector entrepreneurship and investment, this can reduce the need for public resources, which can then be used to improve access and quality of public health care services for the local population. In this sense, trade in health services can result in positive redistribution of scarce public health care resources. Domestic consumers also make gains in terms of better access to affordable quality health care.

Trade in health services through foreign investment may have a positive effect on health service delivery, by improving the management, quality, and cost-effectiveness of services. Increased commercial presence in the health sector is thought to lead to increased competition and greater efficiency, as well as bring in new skills and technology.Trade in health services through temporary migration of health personnel can contribute to national income through remittances. In addition, this form of trade facilitates upgrading of health professional skills.

Negative Impacts

The benefits of trade in health services need to be balanced against potential negative impacts.

Market Imperfections

Trade in health services is likely to be different from trade in other services and trade in commodities for several reasons. One of the fundamental principles underlying free trade is that increased competition will be better for the consumer in terms of lower prices, greater access, higher quality, and efficiency of provision. This principle stems from the notion of perfect competition which is based on:

— perfect information;

— large numbers of buyers and sellers; and

— no barriers to entry and exit in the market.

Price is a signal for buyers and sellers to exchange goods and services. However, the market for health services is highly imperfect, so that increased competition in this market will not necessarily lead to improvements in efficiency, equity, or quality.

While there may be many buyers of health services, the number of suppliers is limited. Public health care systems used to be sole providers of medical services in most developing countries, but these systems were immensely bureaucratic and non-responsive to market forces. With the advent of health care reform, private participation in health care delivery and financing is playing a greater role. While one expects private provision of services to be more efficient, access to care may be curtailed because of inability to pay for services. Quality of care may be affected as there are few regulations and controls within the health sector.

There are many barriers to entry and exit in the health care market. Hospitals are expensive to build and operate, so that there will be few investors in developing countries able to raise sufficient capital. Hospitals in both the public and private sectors have tended to operate as if they had monopoly power. Medical associations often control how many and who gets to practice medicine, which limits entry into the market. In some developing countries, however, there is "overproduction" of health professionals which tends to distort the structure of human capital formation and boost health care costs.

In addition, there is a great deal of uncertainty in the health care marketplace: professionals cannot guarantee a medical outcome, as the effectiveness of treatment is often case-specific. Medical professionals deal with probabilities of outcomes, which implies a certain degree of risk. Consumers often do not have enough information to make informed choices about the best quality and quantity of care. In this context, physicians often act as "agents" for the patient in medical decision-making. In some countries, this phenomenon can lead to escalating costs of care.

Moreover, there is a great deal of asymmetry of information in the health care market between buyer and seller. Patients know their own health status better than insurers, which tends to lead to a condition known as *adverse selection*: sicker individuals tend to join health insurance pools, which eventually drives up the cost of insurance. Higher premiums crowd out certain population groups, leading to additional price distortions in the health insurance market. On the other hand, private health insurers may "cream skim" by selecting only the healthiest patients in the population, to cut costs and secure profits.

There are a large number of positive and negative externalities in the health care market. An externality is a phenomenon which leads to over- or under-consumption of the socially optimal amount of a good or service. This results in inefficiencies and inequities in the marketplace. A classic example of a positive externality is the benefit that accrues to a group of people with the immunization of one person. As more and more people are immunized against a disease, this act tends to protect the population from outbreaks, so that the unimmunized are protected by the actions of the immunized. In this scenario, there is an incentive for people to remain unimmunized.

Therefore, policy makers need to bear in mind that health services have certain unique characteristics which will affect the quantity of services provided and consumed in the global market place. Changing the incentives of providers and consumers will alter health care seeking behaviour, and have implications for free trade.

Crowding out

There is consensus that equity is an important social goal and public health services are an essential input into achieving that objective. Developing countries have endeavoured to provide good quality health care services, either free of charge or at highly subsidized prices to their populations. Some policy makers are concerned that by providing health services to visitors, scarce public resources will be reallocated away from much needed public health programs. The local population will not be provided with access to quality health services.

Crowding out can only occur when public funds are used to develop trade in health services. However, government's role could be to encourage and monitor private sector development of health services that could be traded on the international market. These two tracks for health services can be developed simultaneously, and in a mutually reinforcing way.

NATURE OF HEALTH TOURISM

The recurring question posed in every country is "What is meant by health tourism?" Even for those agencies that have been involved with either promotion or delivery of health tourism activity, there is a growing awareness that there is a lot more to this label and to the development of these 'products' it is not merely an issue of marketing. In the trade context, health tourism is what people are comfortable talking about that is the movement of customers for the consumption of the service in the host country. Within this mode, a range of 'health' services are being provided or traded which for simplicity of discussion can be categorized into three product groups, using the broadest definition of health (rather than medical):

— Wellness/Promotive Care
— Treatment
— Rehabilitation

Table 2 gives the range of products by category that is being considered as feasible in the short and long term for health tourism, many of which are already being provided to visiting patients.

Wellness services are being provided primarily through the tourism industry, and clearly demonstrate the capacity of the countries to support the movement of persons for the consumption of services as well as the growing demand particularly for more healthy and active style vacations. These services tend to be the most highly developed aspect of trade in health services in the region both in terms of product definition and marketing. As such, it has begun to attract the interest of health providers, for example in the provision of complementary healing and herbal medicines.

Table 2. List of Healthcare products/services currently being traded

Wellness	*Treatment*	*Rehabilitation*
i. Spas	i. Elective surgery	i. Dialysis
ii. Lifestyle/Healthy vacations	ii. Cosmetic surgery	ii. Addiction programmes
iii. Nature tourism	iii. Joint replacement	iii. Elderly care programmes
iv. Ecotourism	iv. Cardiothoracic services	
v. Community Tourism	v. Eye surgery	
vi. Resorts	vi. Diagnostic services	
vii. Herbal Treatments	viii. Cancer treatment	
viii. Complementary Healing		

Services in the treatment and rehabilitation categories are being provided primarily through existing health services as an extension of the capacity and interest of the local market. Only a limited number of these services have been developed for the tourist market. Most of the activity is in the private sector, although the public hospitals are also providing care to non-nationals usually on a government-to-government basis. Facilities have been purposely built to attract foreign patients.

Treatment and rehabilitation services are usually considered local services used by tourists, and are not strictly considered as part of health tourism. They however, represent a growing and important input for the continued development of health tourism. In addition, the risks associated with eco-tourism and adventure tourism as more active products compared to the sun, sea and surf packages also put additional demands on the quality of health services to manage emergency interventions. The diversification of the tourism product therefore is calling for a more structured approach to the planning of health services as part of the supporting infrastructure that will be required for a sustainable asset based tourism industry.

The main difference between treatment and rehabilitation services is in the acuteness of the condition which in turn affects the length of time needed for direct interaction with a health provider and the range of services needed for the delivery of a quality service.

Treatment services for which clients will travel will be characterised by relatively predictable shorter time needed with the provider but a broader, more sophisticated range of services; whereas rehabilitation services usually require a longer time to reach a desired outcome and a narrower spectrum of support services.

Planning for Health Tourism

Much of the feasibility of health tourism stems from the growing recognition that health is big business with estimated annual global healthcare expenditure in excess of $3 trillion per annum. Increasingly the industry is being globalized and the factors that may be contributing to the increasing demand for services outside of the country of origin include:

— Increasing costs of services;

— Lack of availability of services due to rationing or regulation;

— An upwardly and outwardly mobile client group;

Movement of clients from less to more sophisticated markets has dominated trade in health services. However, there is no formal collation of data about the movement of persons for health care, either in the country of origin or destination.

Where it is assumed that the main driver is the lack of those services in the country of origin, other reasons include confidence in local services, confidentiality and privacy, lack of diagnostic capacity and in some cases the service is more accessible in terms of cost and other social barriers in a bigger centre. It should not be taken for granted therefore that investment in better infrastructure, without the upgrading in the quality of staff and management will necessarily result in 'import substitution' or keeping the business in the country.

When planning on a country basis, one approach is to look at population, disease, utilisation, economic and social trends and patterns, and model against international standards of good practice in order to take into consideration impact of new approaches on future needs. Models applied to health tourism could use this data to give an indication of the size of potential markets, but the real questions are:

— What is the source of this data and the relevance (or quality) in terms of estimation of demand for health tourism services?

- What segments of this population with a particular health need are willing and able to seek care outside of their country?
- What are the determining factors to ensure a favourable outcome for the client?
- What level of investment is required for that outcome and what proportion of that population segment will be able to attract?
- Is this a profitable business in the long term, given the high level of investment required; or is the investment justified for the viability of the tourism industry and therefore should be cross-subsidized by the tourism sector?

Sources of this type of data would be from surveys looking at health seeking behaviour and preferences. However, a fairly large sample size would be required to capture meaningful information about those who sought care or would be willing to seek care outside their own community and country.

Another approach is to examine tourism statistics, but generally the factors that determine the choice of destination for a vacation and the profile of the tourist coming would be quite different than those for health tourism. Further, the big increase in tourist arrivals in the region in the last 3-4 years has been from cruise ships. The nature of this business is quite different to the stay over arrivals and probably has even less implication for the development of health tourism However, tourism trends can indicate how successful the marketing strategy has been in terms of raising the profile of the country and generally the capacity of the country to move people into and around to access services.

In practice, planning in the health market is heavily influenced by supplier-driven and supplier-induced factors. For example, the biggest increase in activity is usually seen when a new specialist or a new piece of equipment (owned by a specialist) is introduced in the marketplace. Although there is much interest in improving the demand side of the equation, the asymmetry of knowledge and the role of the doctor in prescribing the care regime does not easily lend itself to creating an informed and knowledgeable purchaser when it comes to personal medical need. Most of the success in improving how care is purchased has been through the developments in managed care and strengthening of referral networks.

More success has been achieved with increasing consumer knowledge with respect to the healthy lifestyle approach and this trend is manifested in the increasing interest in fitness, health spas, healthy eating, complementary healing, use of natural herbs for medical treatment, healthy active vacations and in a more interventionist way, cosmetic surgery. In addition, the move to sustainable tourism approaches, and an asset-based tourist product development is resulting in an increased level of activity in Eco Tourism and Adventure Tourism as complementary to the traditional sun, surf and sand product. Natural and complementary healing practices are logical adjuncts to these tourism products.

The nature of this demand is clearly demonstrated by the rapid growth of fitness activities in the larger tourist hotels, the increasing number of spa offerings and the increasing networking of smaller hotels with local fitness and sport businesses. The growth in the treatment and rehabilitation categories has been less remarkable, although there seems to be an increasing number of practitioners treating visitors routinely. The latter service is usually in addition to the normal caseload rather than a specific service developed and targeted to attract tourists. This sense of increased activity is probably therefore a result of the general growth of the private sector and the private sector's interest in looking for populations who can afford to pay for health care.

Many policies and practices do not favour generating business from foreign markets as generally doctors are not allowed by the rules of the profession to actively market themselves or solicit business. The situation is further complicated as most private health facilities are doctor-owned and managed. So whereas there is an increasing number of self-referral for care, most of the business in the health services is based on provider referral and/or recommendation either in the form of formal and informal networks.

The growth of health tourism should be done so as to capitalize on the assets upon which the tourism industry and other services are built i.e. proximity and access to the target markets, relatively strong intellectual capital, an established hospitality industry, and ambient environment. However, the high unit costs of the health service product (due to our small economies of scale) plus the relatively high priced tourism product preclude the region from being price competitive. It would imply a focus on the development of medical services that compete on quality and on market niches for which the client did not put price as one of the key considerations in the decision making, as for example, cosmetic surgery. So based on a supplier driven approach to assessing demand for health tourism services, the emphasis tends to be less on estimating health need and best value for money, but rather more on determining:

- Who are the providers?
- What is their capacity?
- Who is willing to pay for the service?
- Creation and establishment of the product;
- Access to the product through limited direct marketing; and
- Indirect marketing through building of referral networks and a satisfied population.

More action is needed on market surveys in developed markets about health-seeking behaviour to understand why clients would leave their own country and realistically determining if the cost of setting up the service for this client group is justified in terms of the potential return. The main question about south-south trade is the pricing structure of the product and the ability to compete with other developing markets, for those clients truly able to pay.

Barriers to the Trade in Health Services

There are several barriers to the development of trade in health services in general. These are:

- *Nature of medical practice*: Most health care services are provided on a referral basis with the physician acting as a gatekeeper. Practitioners will not want to lose patients, and patients may not be at ease seeking care in unfamiliar surroundings.

  The most important barrier to trade is the emotional security of ill persons, in that they will be in unfamiliar surroundings, far from friends and family. Trade in this type of health service will need to overcome this particular barrier through promotion of quality care and access to interpersonal links through telecommunications, and the like;

— *Laws and regulations*: Clauses contained in laws, regulations and the like, may restrict or block access to the market or discriminate against foreign services or service providers as compared to national ones. The lack of availability of reliable information on government policies and regulations relating to trade in health services represents a significant barrier to trade.

  Three types of legislation appear to affect the supply and demand of medical and health services. These include:

  — qualification and licensing requirements for individual health professionals, including paramedical health professionals;

  — approval requirements for institutional suppliers such as clinics and hospitals; and,

  — rules and practices governing reimbursement under mandatory public or private insurance schemes;

— *Financing of care and insurance coverage*: Portability of health insurance represents a significant barrier to free trade in health services. In most cases, private health insurance policies and public systems do not cover treatment abroad, except in the case of emergency. The portability of health insurance is primarily an issue for the U.S. market, as patients from the UK are covered under national health insurance scheme, and Canada covers all costs of medical care for its citizens. Some European countries offer national health insurance as well.

  Americans older than 65 are eligible for a government-sponsored program (Medicare) to cover hospitalization and other medical costs. Entitlement to Medicare is based on age and working status. Medicare does not cover any care received outside of the country. Another U.S. government program, Medicaid, is for the medically indigent population and those suffering from certain illnesses. Medicaid also does not cover care received outside of the country;

— *Accreditation and standards*: Existing facilities and services cannot provide good quality and reliable backup necessary for trade in health services. The perception of lower quality services will be difficult to overcome without aggressive marketing and upgrading of facilities.

— *Immigration and foreign exchange requirements*: While some countries have changed their immigration legislation to allow for temporary entry of certain categories of health personnel, other restrictions, such as economic needs test requirements; discriminatory licensing procedures; difficulties with accreditation or recognition of foreign professional qualifications; nationality and residency requirements; state and provincial requirements; access to examinations for completion of qualifications; foreign exchange controls; or discriminatory regulation of fees and expenses, may apply.

— *Lack of market research on demand for health services*: Need to increase access to data on demand for health services for potential entrepreneurs and government agencies.

— *Competition within the Region*: Several Latin American countries already have well-established health tourism industries. For instance, direct patient care is a major export of Costa Rica, Cuba, Colombia, and Mexico

Health Service Trade: Case of English-speaking Caribbean

Health tourism thrives in islands with an expanding and booming tourism industry and a culture and economy that is geared to looking at tourist markets. The Bahamas is a good case in point where there are a range of health tourism activities associated with the turnaround in tourism in the last few years that has resulted from a surge of FDI. By way of comparison, Dominica has been active in developing its tourism industry over the last 10 years recording a significant increase in arrivals in the last 2 years due to cruise ship visitors. The number of stay-over visitors has however, stagnated, and that occupancy rates in many of the hotels the smaller ones are not high. Some of the constraints to the development of the stay-over tourism industry in Dominica will also constraint the development of health tourism. The relationship between tourism and health services can also be frustrated where the health services are weak and distant from the tourist resorts as in Jamaica.

The English-speaking Caribbean has many characteristics that could facilitate successful development of health tourism. These include attractive climate and environment; well-trained health practitioners; reliable telecommunications and good transport infrastructure; excellent hotel and tourism services; an educated population; and, lower labour costs than most developed countries.

Previous studies have emphasized that the greatest returns in the Caribbean will stem from development of health tourism; health resorts and spas integrating complementary and alternative medicine; cosmetic surgery; rehabilitation; and convalescent care.

Trade in health services may be more successful with the U.S. market than with the Canadian, European, or South American market because it has a large uninsured and underinsured population, as well as higher prices of medical care. Geographical proximity also makes this market more attractive. In Canada, the de-listing of certain services from the national health system may represent some opportunities for health tourism in the Caribbean in the future.

However, the competitiveness of the Region's health services will depend upon the price, availability of skilled professionals, service differentiation, and availability of necessary technology and facilities.

There are several worldwide trends that could possibly generate market opportunities for the English-speaking Caribbean for trade in health services, including the:

— aging of the population and resultant increases in demand for cosmetic surgery, spas, and retirement communities;

— growing affluence of the younger population, particularly in the U.S.;

— lifestyles in Europe and North America which put a premium on vacations which can offer spa facilities, fitness, or addiction treatment; and,

— growth in lifestyle -related illnesses and health problems, such as chronic conditions.

There appears to be a growing interest and activity in the development of spas and complementary healing practices in response to increased demand from the international marketplace. However, much of the development has remained relatively fragmented, small scale with most of the progress in the range of wellness services located in the tourism infrastructure.

Health Tourism Services

Convalescent and Elder Care

Convalescent and elder care is one area that is receiving growing attention vis-a-vis trade in health services. This is because of the rapidly aging world population, which is leading to growing numbers of elderly. The senior population accounts for 25.5% of the population of the UK; 20.9% of the U.S. population, and 28.4% of the German population. The average disposable income of three million retired people in the OECD countries ranges from U.S.$12,000 to U.S.$20,000 per year. While some seniors being fairly well off, and others struggling to live below the poverty line, there is a sizeable senior population that has the ability to finance travel. Seniors (persons older than 50 years of age) accounted 18% of all visits abroad in 1996, and the number of long haul trips has increased to nearly 500,000 in the same year. In the U.S., seniors account for one-fifth of the population, but represent almost half of the long-haul trips. The senior's travel market (aged 55 years or older) exceeds 100 million, and accounts for one in six international trips.

Persons aged 60 years or older accounted for nearly 10% of total arrivals to the Caribbean in 1998. Forty-six percent of all arrivals were for persons aged 40 years and older. In Barbados, senior arrivals have been increasing steadily since 1989, representing 29% of total arrivals in 1998. Senior travellers to the Caribbean represent a niche market that cannot be overemphasised. Health tourism which is designed around the needs of seniors may be a successful enterprise for the Region.

Prior to major volcanic activity on Montserrat, the island had an expatriate community of nearly 10% of the population. Approximately 45% of retirees came from Canada, 45% from the northeastern United States, and 10% from the United Kingdom. Most of the retirees were wealthy who wanted the reprieve of life on a tropical island. Residency of retirees created demand for both skilled and unskilled labour, including maids, gardeners, and construction workers. Efforts were made to integrate the retirement community into Montserrat.

Unfortunately, health issues were cited as the primary reason for leaving the retirement community. Retirees felt that the local health system was inadequate for their needs. While payment for health care on Montserrat was not a problem for this population group, those coming from the U.S. were not eligible for health care coverage under their insurance plans.

Other reasons for leaving the island included being far away from family and friends, and financial considerations. Although this population group was wealthy, unexpected changes in the cost of living would affect the cost-effectiveness of staying in Montserrat. Bureaucratic procedures, such as those pertaining to work permits, alien-landholding acts, and visas created disincentives for the community to remain on the island.

Anguilla has considered attracting the retirement community of Montserrat. There are plans to develop a similar community in Dominica over the next few years by Global Medical Health Centres and Resorts.

In Jamaica there are already systems in place to open the market for retirement communities. Jamaicans repatriating after retirement represent a big market for retirement communities but there are many issues now about their safety and absorption back into their communities.

Another impediment to development of convalescent care in the Caribbean is the potential shortage of skilled nursing staff, with the need to import health professionals in the short-run. In the longer-term, retention of Caribbean health professionals may improve due to greater opportunities within the Region. Growing personal security problems in some countries will inhibit demand for this type of health tourism.

Because of the aging population worldwide, the need for health care services for the elderly is rising. There are a few private nursing homes operating in the region which have, on occasion, offered services to visitors. One of these is the Barbados Home Nursing Agency, which began operation in 1982. This facility provides convalescent care for patients coming out of the Queen Elizabeth Hospital. The facility is staffed by trained nurses with physicians on call. The occupancy rate is approximately 70% in this 18 bed facility, though occupancy is seasonal. On average, patients stay three months in the facility, with six months being the maximum length of stay. Financially, the facility is surviving, though there are very tight margins with this type of service, as the cost of labour and benefits are high. It appears that there is room in Barbados for additional facilities, as competition in this domain is not that great.

Rehabilitation from Drug and Alcohol Dependency

Drug and alcohol dependency services represent another potential growth area for the Caribbean. Several facilities currently exist in the Caribbean: one of which is highly successful on an international scale.

The Crossroads Centre at Willoughby Bay, Antigua is a non-profit, 36-bed residential facility located on 20 acres in the southeast coast of Antigua, with an excellent view of the sea. The 29-day program, based on the Twelve Steps of Alcoholics Anonymous (AA) helps clients recover from alcohol and other dependencies. Crossroads is currently rated third in the world

Other rehabilitation services of this type are available in Antigua and the Caribbean. For instance, the Centre refers patients who require a longer program to Mt. St. Benedict in Trinidad. The Turning Point (St. Lucia) and Charter House are both government run facilities in the Region. In addition, the Mount St. John's Medical Centre in Antigua is under development and will be a 187-bed state of the art hospital catering to local and foreign clientele. It is expected that this hospital will provide medical and support backup to the Centre.

The Centre contributes to the local economy through employment of Antiguan nationals as support personnel, administrative and clerical staff, and clinic professionals. Approximately 90% of the materials and supplies used in the Centre are sourced in Antigua, which also contributes to the economy. Because the families of clients utilize tourist facilities, and the Centre hosts alumni reunions of clients and spouses, other sectors in the economy benefit from the operation of this facility. Nevertheless, because some of the inputs and staff come from outside the country, it is difficult to gauge the net foreign exchange contribution.

One of the major drawbacks is that clients cannot claim insurance for the services provided at Crossroads. Recommendations include opening up of international accreditation, and creation of regional bodies to handle accreditation. Because of the specialized nature of rehabilitative services, and the strong competition which exists for clientele, this type of activity may not have the strongest growth potential for the Caribbean. Other issues, such as the perception of the local population towards the clientele, may also prevent widespread growth of this type of health service in the Region.

This case suggests that while the goal was to provide dependency services to the local population, it was necessary to cultivate an international export market first to generate sufficient resources to subsidize patients from the West Indies. This type of model is potentially replicable in the future.

Health Resorts

Health resorts and spas are popular in North America and Europe as leisure-time activities, particularly as a result of trends toward healthy living, stress reduction, and spiritual rejuvenation. The Caribbean has a comparative advantage because of the natural beauty and resources of the islands. This type of tourism can be linked to resorts and hotels that offer holistic health treatment, such as aromatherapy, yoga, fitness and exercise programs, weight loss and nutrition counselling, and other types of spa treatments. There are few resorts in the Caribbean developed for the purpose of providing stress reduction, and this represents a major potential growth area for Caribbean tourism, given the growing interest in healthy lifestyles and alternative and complementary medicine worldwide.

While many hotels in the region have added fitness and day spa services for their clients, there are few resorts in the Caribbean which have been developed solely for the purpose of providing a retreat atmosphere for stress reduction and alternative healing. For instance, analysis of information suggests that there are less than 30 full-service health spas operating in the English-speaking CARICOM countries, out of a total of 545 advertisements placed, which is less than 5% of hotels and resorts.

Presently, a number of hotels provide fitness and day spa services, such as facials and massage therapy. La Source in Grenada, Le Sport in St. Lucia, Sandy Lane in Barbados, and most of the Sandals Resorts offer specialized spa and wellness services. In the Bahamas four of the major hotels have spa services and one hotel, the Yoga Retreat on Paradise Island offers a resort package based on complementary healing and a high return visitor rate.

Very few hotels have been designed which incorporate alternative healing in a spa facility. One exception is Sandy Lane Hotel which is being renovated to include a three-story, 45,000 square foot spa facility with 11 VIP suites. Services to be provided include: hydrotherapy, massage, aromatherapy, ayurvedic treatments, thalassotherapy, among others. Spa services will be a la carte in terms of pricing. Therapists will be mainly from Barbados who have undergone an eight-week training session, with continuing training throughout their employment. Physician and physiotherapy services will be available on-call.

Sandy Lane is marketed as a hotel with a spa. They expect their guests to come primarily from the U.K., Europe and the U.S. In fact, they hope the spa will help develop the American market for the hotel. Managers feel there is little competition for their spa services within the Caribbean. The spa is modelled on other international resorts and spas, such as the Oriental Hotel in Bangkok, and is expected to attract this type of clientele.

Because this type of facility is new to Barbados, Sandy Lane has found the government very keen to assist in its development. One drawback has been the superficiality of some of the training courses in massage and aesthetics offered on the island. There is need for upgrading of these courses, as well as to provide certification. Management believes that licensing and regulation of these types of practitioners will only strengthen this type of tourism product in Barbados.

There are several smaller establishments providing alternative and complementary medicine and healing in Barbados, and a few of them advertise directly to tourists. Examples include the Caribbean Stress Management Institute, St. John; Windward Natural Health, St. James; The Integrated Natural Health Shoppe and Clinic, Hastings; and Reiki School of Natural Healing. In addition, there is a wide range of alternative and complementary practitioners on the island who offer Reiki, acupuncture, homeopathy, massage therapy, aromatherapy, and iridology, among others.

Based in Barbados, the Caribbean Association of Complementary and Alternative Medicine (CACAM) is a professional Caribbean association of alternative and complementary practitioners, groups and organizations. The purpose of CACAM is to ensure the integration, acceptance and expansion of alternative and complementary medicine within the health care system through professional and public education; development of practice standards, and advocacy and research.

CACAM supports alternative and complementary medicine practice in the areas of acupuncture/ acupressure, aromatherapy, Chinese medicine, chiropractic medicine, homeopathy, massage therapy, nutrition, polarity therapy, Reiki, and yoga, among others. The organization was started at the end of 1998, and has approximately 35 members. CACAM hosts a popular annual symposium on alternative and complementary medicine in Barbados.

Alternative and complementary practitioners have trained themselves at their own expense, and represent a tremendous, yet untapped, human resource in the Region. CACAM and its members represent a possible resource for resort operators to tap into in establishing holistic health and spa treatments.

The World Health Assembly, under WHA 30.49 urges governments to give adequate importance to traditional or alternative systems of medicine. This policy is in response to growing demand for complementary medicine worldwide, particularly among the U.S. population. Provision of alternative and complementary health services represents a potential niche market for the English-speaking Caribbean.

A recent study found that the proportion of U.S. adults who used at least one alternative therapy increased from 33% to 42% between 1990 and 1997, resulting in a rise from 427 million visits to 629 million visits for alternative therapies per year. Alternative therapies were used most for chronic conditions. The study also found an increase in expenditure from $14.6 billion to $21 billion. Insurance coverage did not change over this period, so the increased expenditure comes largely from out-of-pocket.

Another study finds that Europeans have a tradition of visiting health resorts and spas. The largest market for health tourism is Germany, followed by Italy and France, particularly for spa treatments and health resorts. Thalassotherapy (sea water treatment) and thermal resorts have the greatest growth potential in Europe.

With today's growing enthusiasm for health and fitness, spas and health resorts should be able to tap a receptive market of younger, higher income clients who are willing to pay for a holiday that reduces stress and includes pampering. The key will be in marketing services once they have been developed.

The Ministry of Health in Barbados is aware of the proliferation of paramedical practitioners in Barbados, as well as the growing use of alternative medicine by the Barbadian population and visitors. There is a well-received, call-in radio show hosted by one of the island's alternative practitioners. The Ministry of Health has established the Paramedical Professions Council to establish standards of operation for alternative systems of medicine in the country, and to provide for registration of professions supplementary to the Conventional Medicine. However, there is currently no licensing or registration in operation. Practitioners are interested in legislation which would integrate them more into the mainstream of health care in Barbados.

Dominica boasts of a strong tradition of herbal medicines and traditional healing practices and lays claim to the oldest living person in the world. Nature tourism and eco tourism have been available in Dominica before it was fashionable and the country is interested in moving forward with that and the marketing of their natural spas the sulphur springs which traditionally have been known for their healing properties.

Cosmetic Surgery

The aging of the population and the growing affluence of some population segments, such as the baby boomers, represent potential market niches for provision of cosmetic surgery. Cosmetic surgery has been provided on Tortola in BVI since the mid-1970s. The market for these services is approximately 50% Caribbean; 40% North American; and 10% from Europe. Puerto Rico also offers plastic surgery, but does not appear to be competing in the same market. Other islands, such as Barbados also offer cosmetic surgery to foreign visitors. Some services are also provided by Tapion in St. Lucia and in Trinidad and Tobago to a clientele primarily from the Caribbean.

A small 12 bed hospital in Lyford Cay in The Bahamas has a cosmetic surgery service geared to tourists, and is considered quite exclusive by virtue of price and reputation. No active marketing is done of the service, which indicates that clients are offered this option by the surgeons involved with Lyford Cay as part of their practice in the USA. There is resident staff in the hospital, and locals are known to go there for routine care. There is one primary cosmetic surgeon on the island who performs breast reduction, liposuction, and abdominal plasty. Patients come from the U.S., the UK, and other Caribbean countries.

Given how tightly regulated the physician market is in Barbados, it is unlikely that this is an area which will be easily expanded in the future Growing demand for plastic surgery will be a positive factor for trade in this area for the future. However, this type of service can only be successful on a larger scale in the Caribbean if a quality product is provided at a lower cost to the patient. In addition, emergency medical backup must be available for effective care and treatment. Confidentiality of the services will be an important factor for success.

Telemedicine and Cross-border Trade

Within the English-speaking Caribbean, telemedicine has many applications for improving the access of the local population to health care, while at the same time providing continuing education and training opportunities for health professionals. Currently, there is a relationship between medical practitioners in St. Kitts and Dalhousie University, Canada for radiographic services.

Telemedicine is a computer-based technology, which can assist in providing services which are not locally available, or to treat patients in rural areas through more cost-effective home-base care. The difficulty for the Caribbean in using this technology is related to the cost of establishing and maintaining the system. A centralized telemedicine link costs between $25,000 to $50,000, depending upon the type of technology. However, home-based units, which may be ideal for inter-island consultation and communication, cost $5,000 with a central monitoring facility costing approximately $7,500. The viability of this option will be improved if a mechanism can be developed within the Region to share the costs and benefits of such a service.

Telemedicine is currently not available in Barbados. The MOH believes this is not a viable option for health tourism as many practitioners and MOH personnel do not have access to computers, nor are they particularly computer literate.

Other Health Services

Curative health tourism focuses on providing treatment, diagnostic care, or surgical care to patients who travel from their own country. Barbados is able to provide health care services to visitors through its well-developed health sector, comprised of a system of polyclinics, district hospitals, and the Queen Elizabeth Hospital in the public sector, which serves as a referral hospital for the Eastern Caribbean. Approximately 150 private physicians also practice in the country. The private sector also includes private emergency clinics and ambulance services, laboratories and diagnostic services, and a private hospital. Bayview Hospital regularly supplies health services for cruise line passengers through contract arrangements with cruise line operators, such as Goddard Shipping and DaCosta Shipping. In fact, cruise line operators are so confident in the medical services provided in Barbados, that they often hold passengers on ship until they arrive in Barbados for medical attention.

Other health services have developed for use of tourists while on the islands including dialysis services, herbal treatments and the private hospital group, Doctor's Hospital in The Bahamas reports that about 15% of its caseload is geared towards tourists seeking care during their visit. The public sector facilities do not feel that tourists use their facilities to any great extent, as most of their specialists also have private offices outside of either Princess Margaret Hospital or Doctor's hospital.

Since the late 1980s and early 1990s the Government of Trinidad and Tobago had embarked on initiatives to encourage the sharing of health services with neighbouring islands provided by the Eric Williams Medical Sciences Complex (EWMSC). However, EWMSC is still not fully commissioned and therefore has operational constraints in openly marketing itself to the region. It does provide care to individuals from Guyana, Grenada, St. Kitts, St Lucia and Barbados on a self referral basis or on a government referral. The link is usually by referring physician. The operational constraints of EWMSC are related to the ambiguity of the employment status of the staff who work there, and the inability of the government to fund the proper start up of the facility. For EWMSC to be a centre of excellence for hospital services, it must provide a full range of support services including the basic hospital specialities before it can provide in a competitive way tertiary or sub-specialities, which in turn can be marketed on the export market. Much of the referral now is done in the same pattern of utilisation that exists in the private sector throughout the Caribbean, on a piecemeal basis but without the proper support framework if the patient becomes complicated.

EWMSC offers a cardiology service in a joint venture arrangement with a local company who in turn works collaboratively with a European partner. When the programme is started, the cardiothoracic surgeon would come down on a regular basis to do cases that were booked and evaluated by the local team. In recent years, the programme has suffered from the loss of nursing staff for immediate post operative care, so now the visiting team also comprises 1 or 2 cardiac intensive care nurses who remain for about 2-5 days after the operation. Some training is also being provided to local nurses. A similar interventionist service is also being provided in a private hospital in the North with a surgeon from the USA, and there are plans for the construction of a new facility specializing in cardiac treatment.

The Complex has also tried over the years to negotiate a contract with an international partner to set up radiotherapy services as the National Health Plan calls for the transfer of radiotherapy services and the establishment of a cancer treatment centre at Mt. Hope. However, this has not been successful because of the lack of the ability of EWMSC to complete the negotiation in time and/or to properly evaluate the international partner. Coincidentally, the North West RHA has negotiated a CT Scan service at Port of Spain General Hospital in a joint venture arrangement with Atlantic Medical.

The private sector anecdotally reports seeing foreign patients on a fairly regular basis, primarily in the sub specialities ophthalmology, cosmetic surgery, orthopaedics the majority of which are from Guyana, Grenada and Antigua. Like the foreign patients who go to EWMSC, there is no active marketing being done, but most patients self refer (because of personal reference) or is sent by a referring physician. Most of the private facilities are owned by doctors. EWMSC management speculates that this could be one of the contributing reasons why to date the Complex remains uncommissioned although the doctors would argue that is purely bad design and planning. The MoH collates some data on private sector activity, but is aware that there is a significant level of under reporting and certainly no statistics about treatment of foreign patients.

Role of the Private Sector

In Jamaica the private sector providers have continued on their own to provide and expand where possible their range of services based on information shared on a sense from the workshop of increasing demand in the marketplace. They do not see the equity and affordability issues as their concern and are focused almost exclusively on expanding the local market for their services by attracting the international market.

Distinct from any other private provider in the Caribbean, Doctor's Hospital is actively engaged in providing care to tourists, has embarked on the development of a health insurance product, and is presently commissioning an ambulatory centre and wellness product in affiliation with an internationally recognized fitness agency to specifically target vacationers looking for a fitness oriented holiday complete with medical assessment and support and looking at linking their facilities with telemedicine links. They would be willing to consider extending the network to the family islands and will have a link to the USA.

Trade Issues

In general, the Ministries of Foreign Affairs and International Trade have not been active participants on any of the recent round of health tourism initiatives. The focus to date has been broadly on intra-regional trade and negotiating liberalization of the CARICOM market and there has been no detailed look at trade in health services specifically.

Broader trade negotiations will have potential effects on trade in health services. As regards the movement of consumers, Governments are keen to look at the management of health risks both in terms of communicable diseases but also if there was risk of decreased access to health care as a result either through an increase in price or loss of local labour.

The movement of professionals is a priority area for liberalization as this would allow easier movement for training and upgrading of skills, but would need to explore incremental liberalization in terms of health as it relates to mutual recognition. Most Caribbean countries import and export health professionals. They have to be careful not to distort the local labour market so there is a need to look at the movement of labour into the country to support these offshore medical centres

Foreign investment contributes to the capacity to manage quality of care for research and experimental care programmes. As a rule, the Caribbean is a less regulated environment than the US and Europe, therefore needs to be affiliated with a reputable programme or facility. The services provided by foreign investors must benefit the local population by stimulating the quality of the local health services.

Island Dialysis is one of the few examples of direct foreign investment in health in Barbados. This facility is operated by the Atlantic Healthcare Group, Inc. out of Ontario, Canada, which also runs similar facilities in Jamaica, St. Lucia, and Puerto Rico. The facility began operation in Barbados two years ago, and employs local staff of four nurses, with two physicians who act as consultants to the facility. While they cater primarily to tourists, they have six local clients. They average approximately 30 clients per month and have 10 dialysis machines. The company advertises its services in several trade magazines, and has a website with links to tourist facilities, information about each Caribbean island, and support services. Patients are charged \$320 per treatment for a less than three-week period; \$290 for more than a three week period; and \$280 for more than five weeks. A deposit of \$640 is required to secure a dialysis spot.

In some countries such as Barbados, the MOH is not formally involved in the application and approval process of foreign direct investment for health services in the country. In Barbados investors interested to develop a health facility or practice can do so without MOH approval, by working through the Chamber of Commerce, the Barbados IDC, and the Office of Economic Affairs.

Public Policy and Health Tourism

In most CARICOM countries, there is presently no government strategy to include trade in health services as part of economic development. The MoH is not actively involved in specific initiatives on health tourism or trade in health services issues. The focus tends to be in the implementation of the Health Sector Reform Programme which aims to improve the quality of health services available to the population and using the strategy of the separation of the government's provider function from its 'purchasing' function.

In Jamaica, for example, MoH's orientation has primarily been on raising the public health standards of the hotel industry and so to safeguard the visitors' health while in Jamaica. The Health Sector Reform Programme has not considered health tourism as a specific issue although developing public -private partnerships falls under the Policy and Planning Division. Ministry of Tourism has been focused on developing the sustainable tourism strategy that could have implications for health tourism.

In Trinidad and Tobago, from the MoH's perspective, work has been ongoing in the Directorate of Quality Management in the development of a quality framework including new legislation, licensing and accreditation issues and establishing mechanisms for monitoring customer satisfaction. The Health Services Act has been drafted to replace the current Hospitals Act and to establish the framework for monitoring quality in all health facilities, including laboratories, diagnostic centres, outpatient clinics and day surgery centres which have been growing in an unregulated fashion to date. Both RHA and private facilities will be governed by this law. Work is also needed to modernize the Public Health Act and for improving professional self regulation.

Strategy for Trade in Health Tourism Services

There are serious lessons to be learnt from the literature and on globalisation and tourism and financial services industries in terms of government not being able to play their appropriate role in policy, regulation and consumer protection. Whereas it may seem obvious that the private sector is the 'engine of growth' of trade, the Government must provide a stewardship role in ensuring equity, quality, and sustainable development. It is important therefore that the strategy addresses the weaknesses in both the public and private sectors, and aim for balanced development of appropriate structures and instruments suitable to the business of trade in health services.

The lessons from the last decade of globalisation and implications for small developing countries can be applied to the issues of trade in health services. Small developing economies differ from other economies in structural characteristics which have implications for the character of the growth process and the capacity for adjustment and include:

— Economic vulnerability because export concentration on a few primary commodities, a high trade/GDP ratio or degree of openness and their small size
— Income volatility due to susceptibility to natural disasters, export instability, higher risk ratings for FDI and constrained adjustment capacity (structural rigidities and institutional weaknesses)
— Lack of international competitiveness due to constraints on material and labour inputs mainly because of the small economy of scale and higher transportation costs which lead to a higher unit production cost.

Small countries can gain from openness if they have the adaptive capacity to adjust and seize the opportunities given the characteristics outlined above. The world economy continues to change at an exponential rate. Those countries that respond to these changes by focusing on protectionist policies are not expected to achieve growth as it is not possible to insulate production or demand from global competition this is evident in the health sector by the Caribbean's continued loss of critical skilled labour in nursing and medicine.

There is need for pro-active adjustment and strategic global repositioning in small countries with respect to trade in health services. Such a strategic response must be holistic and implies profound structural transformation and reform. This will involve development of trade, fiscal and credit policies, supported by education and technology initiatives and close collaboration between the government and the business sectors.

Without this strategic approach, it is not likely that the small countries will be able to develop world class health providers capable of effectively competing in the global marketplace. Within this framework, each country will have to decide who would lead the development strategy and be accountable for the development objectives being achieved. This is separate and apart from the actual delivery of the services and does not necessarily have to be the same organization. The potential leaders for the strategy include:

— Ministry of Health
— Ministry of Tourism
— Ministry of Trade
— Development/Investment Authority
— Tourism Development Agency
— Private Sector Agency
— Providers – public or private
— Insurance Industry
— Employers
— Joint Task Force/committees

Figure 1 illustrates these key players and present relationships and groups them into four broad roles: investors, regulators, providers and customers or clients.Each country in moving forward will need to complete a stakeholder analysis of or al least evaluate the various interests, resources and potential problems associated with trade in health tourism to determine the most appropriate role for each player in the formulation and implementation of the development strategy. Figure 1 also attempts to illustrate how the strategy must recognize that the development of activities pertaining to the health tourism industry will both positively and negatively affect the delivery of care for residents of the country (as clients) and this must be a key consideration in moving forward. This is one of the key lessons that is driving the development of sustainable tourism strategies throughout the Region after nearly two decades of tourism development and, therefore should be critical in moving forward into further commercializing what has traditionally been considered a social sector. Good health status of the people is critical to the sustainable economic development of the country. Current or future generations should not be placed at risk by strategies for maximizing income or foreign exchange.

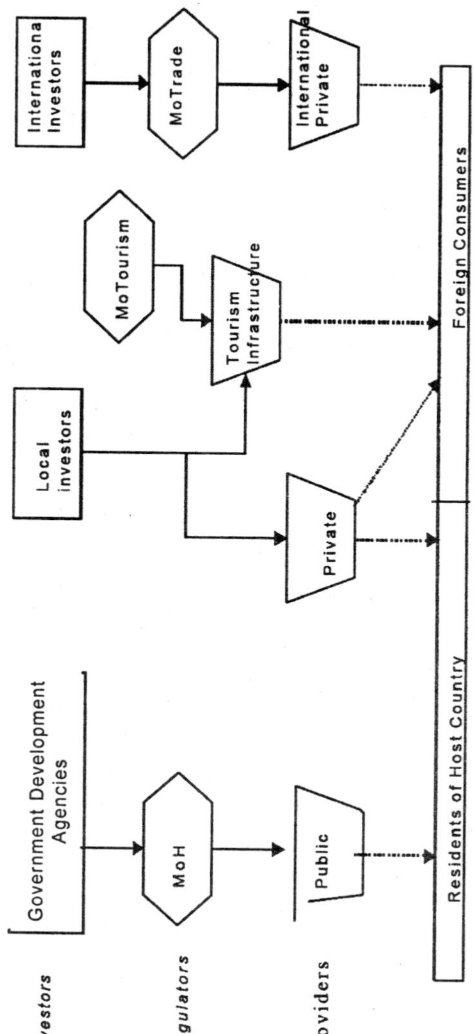

Figure 1. The Key Players and The Relationships in the Health Sector

In addition, the intention should not be to draw boundaries around health care for residents and those for tourists. Rather, the aim should be to improve access as well as quality for the local residents as is done now in seeking care in the local private sector and overseas.

In moving forward with the strategy for health tourism, there is a critical need for the further development of cross linkages, at the three levels of investment, regulation and provision, among:

— sectors (health, tourism, trade);
— public and private;
— national and international.

In the trade and tourism business, this need for promotion and more international focus, led to the development of many of the trade and investment authorities or agencies in the CARICOM e.g. NDC, JAMPRO, TIDCO, BIA to play key roles in marketing and attracting investment. However, many of these agencies now struggle with how to address new sector interests, such as health, and how to affect policy and capacity issues required for implementation of the proposed investment projects. None of these agencies currently have a technical health capacity.

The role of regional agencies involved in trade, tourism and health services will also need to be explored in terms of contributions to common issues of design, development and implementation in collaboration with other national and international agencies and firms. Strengthening of the regional trading of health services could play a useful role in managed liberalization. Regional agencies can act as regulators by creating standards for industry regionally and internationally, including the negotiation of intra-regional trade policies as they affect trade in health services.

The big question still remains how to proactively and pragmatically engage the private sector within a framework of socially agreed objectives. This implies that government should play a stronger role in regulating, monitoring and involving the private sector in service delivery, particularly in relation to the public health goals. An improved policy and regulatory framework is needed to improve the allocation of resources and equity. There is still a fair amount of duplication of local resources, low returns on investment and inadequate cost-effective customer service. Ultimately, this misallocation of resources in the private sector undermines its efficiency and international competitiveness. It exacerbates the inherent weaknesses of small developing countries as they relate to economies of scale, labour inputs and high production costs. The above strategy therefore must involve leadership that can work across traditional boundaries and relationships to position the industry in a way that creates and contributes to a new paradigm of health care.

Building Blocks and Inputs

Figure 2 illustrates some of the key building blocks for the development of the industry or group of services called health tourism, where it is assumed that tourism development will provide many of the inputs, and that the health service (including complementary healing) will itself require health specific inputs in terms of health providers, management, infrastructure and training.

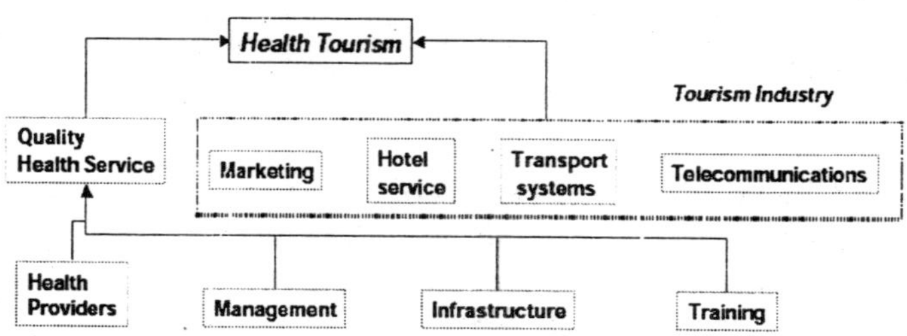

Figure 2. Inputs For The Health Tourism Industry

In terms of the trade relationships, the opportunities through the analysis of the various modes provides an additional development perspective of how trade and globalisation can be enablers to the development of the industry. This is illustrated in Figure 3. If one views trade in health tourism services as essentially the movement of consumers, then some key demand determinants are shown in Figure 3. Others relate to availability, quality, price, distance and cultural and social factors.

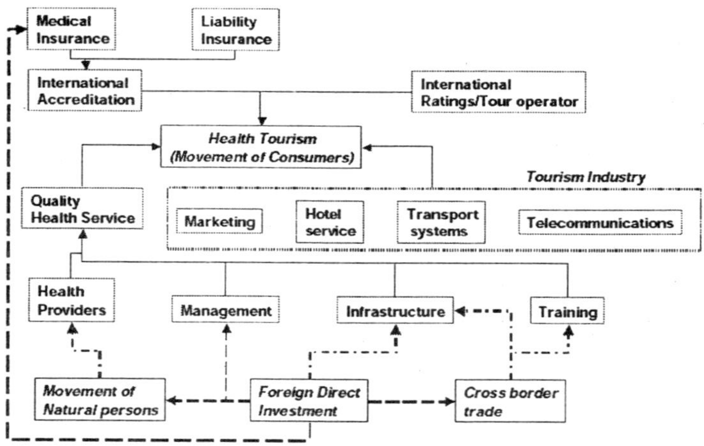

Figure 3. Strategic Framework For Expanding Trade in Health Tourism

Role of Foreign Direct Investment (FDI)

Investment by foreign individuals or companies in the health care arena in a host country is another mode of trade in health services. Foreign investment in the health sector includes facility operation or management. In addition, health insurance companies establishing branch offices overseas represent foreign direct investment. Managed care services, which combine management and insurance into one entity, are another form of trade in the health sector. Many providers of health services have established themselves in foreign countries through joint ventures with local partners.

Foreign investment in the health arena is more prevalent outside of the Caribbean. For instance, sales by U.S. majority-owned health care providers amounted to $US 469 million in 1995. By the mid 1990s, the Singapore-based Parkway Group Healthcare Pte. had acquired several hospitals in Asia and Britain. Some clinics in Canada are trying to exploit the American market. Given the complexities of the health market that FDI be viewed as more than a source of capital funds and international partners be sought to provide the management, technical, infrastructure and training inputs required to develop an internationally competitive service. The links to an international network would also help the country to gain access to the export market (through the referral network) and gain accreditation.

International accreditation will be key to obtaining medical insurance and medical liability coverage. Even if insurance companies developed products that would allow international coverage in the Caribbean, the price of that coverage rises with more freedom of choice both in terms of provider and range of services covered. International accreditation will facilitate Caribbean-based facilities to be part of globally recognized networks of a certain quality and to be properly rated for risks. The opportunity will also be provided to broaden the range of services to more aesthetic ones normally outside of any covered insurance package e.g. cosmetic surgery.

This is not to suggest that one investor needs to provide the whole range of support. It is important that all aspects of this mode of trade be explored in order to address the managerial and technical constraints and weaknesses that presently exist in the health sector, which, in some CARICOM countries, is an even bigger constraint than availability of funds for capital investment.

What needs to be encouraged is real public-private partnership on both the capital and recurrent expenditure issues. The key characteristics of investment in the health sector include:

- High level of investment in infrastructure, systems and people;
- Longer time to realize potential profits because of the nature of the product and the imperfections in the market;
- Lower profit margins or return on investment because high social value of the services gains may not be in the service delivery itself but in downstream products or services;
- Medium to high risk investment requiring tight management throughout the lifetime of the project.

The rapid growth in hotel investment in the Bahamas is related to the large investment in infrastructure. It is also connected to the fact that foreign investors are managing and running the businesses, marketing through the international networks and providing significant amount of training and employment to local residents. This would imply that adequate arrangements for the movement of natural persons are also critical.

Policy, regulatory, institutional and legislative barriers to foreign investment in health Tourism have been highlighted in the region such as uncertainty and lack of transparency concerning work permits, Alien-Landholding Acts, and visas as well as the absence of information on government policies and regulations pertaining to the export of health care services. The lack of a set of formal regulations readily available to interested investors and governing standards for medical care, licensing, quality assurance and control procedures, clinical practice, and facilities operations has been particularly underscored. Policies regarding the licensing and approval of new technologies, treatments, and drugs were also underscored.

Taxes in relation to the purchase of property and the import of high technology medical equipment were also noted as another deterrent of foreign investment Labour laws are also seen as problematic for expatriates. It is difficult to obtain work permits and the uncertainty of renewal makes many foreigners reluctant to invest. In addition, the legal and regulatory constraints are subject to both interpretation and discretion. Approval times also involve a lot of uncertainty.

While countries are making efforts to eliminate these barriers, the question has been raised as to whether it is sufficient to eliminate barriers or is it also necessary to provide incentives? The debate on the granting of incentives to correct market failures has raged over the years without any firm conclusions and guidelines. The conditions under which incentives work or do not work are still not known with any precision.

There is a suggestion that financial incentives matter and are needed in health services. An examination of incentive legislation in the six countries studied indicated that none of them offered special financial incentives for the health services industry but Governments in the region have the inherent right to take "off- the - book" decisions to offer special financial incentives. It is often said in the region that no specific incentives are tailored to any sector de jure even though a range of them exists de facto. The design of financial incentives to address the peculiarities of health sector investment is often suggested as a way to stimulate and manage FDI. Governments have however been advised to stay away from sector-specific incentives that tend to distort investment. A more general industry-neutral approach avoids or reduces special pleading. It is nondiscriminatory and less distortionary. This tendency to discretionary provision of incentives also leads to foreign firms being given more incentives than local firms. Costly competition among Caribbean countries is also a by-product which a cooperative efforts over the years have attempted to prevent but with little success.

In an imperfect world, special incentives never go away, and by far, the greatest competition for investment is among developing countries. The evidence from the Bahamas case study suggests that FDI can make a big difference and is responsive to liberal policies. Bahamas however, offered a range of incentives for hotel investment as laid out in the Hotel Encouragement Act and supporting regulations managed by the Office of the Prime Minister (OPM) through the Bahamas Investment Authority.

In the absence of an agreement among CARICOM countries as well as internationally acceptable conventions to limit unhealthy competition in the granting of incentives, special incentives will continue to stimulate investment in the region. The case of the Bahamas in hotel investment seems to illustrate that in spite of liberal policies to foreign investment that reduced barriers, special incentives were still necessary. The evidence in the health sector is not conclusive enough to suggest that countries could avoid using special sector-specific incentives. Greater emphasis should also be placed on attracting long-term investment as against short-term 'footloose' industries. Lessons learnt from experiences where projects have not achieved the long-term economic objectives but investors have been able to take the short term financial benefits, must be considered seriously in designing the incentive package. The project should be assessed on:

— Clear identification of market demand;
— Technical and managerial capacity to implement the project;
— Financial analysis demonstrating the longer-term feasibility of the venture.

In addition, in the health sector, financial investment incentives should be considered as only part of the total incentive package, in that liability and risk management issues could come up long after the investor has reaped the start-up benefits. Again, as history will show in the health sector, it is easy to build the facility but very difficult to run it. Incentives also could be developed to encourage joint ventures with local partners. Local partners should clearly demonstrate their contribution to the partnership and a capacity to participate actively in the venture. Care needs to be taken so that incentives do not lead to the creation of local medical cartels.

Social Goals and Free Trade

The question of meeting the social goals in the health sector in the context of freer trade and in a search to increase exports of health services must receive greater priority in national policy making. Liberalization of trade (imports or exports) can lead to changes in the prices of certain goods and services and have an impact on access. This is reflected in the concern about crowding out of poor consumers. There is a feeling that provision of medical services for wealthy tourists may "crowd out" provision of quality health care. This is particularly true when considering the limited number of nurses and doctors and various competing interests in this area.

The effect of health tourism may be to aggravate the shift of the labour force away from serving the general public towards more elitist groups and also increasing the demand for more expensive services. The additional costs of establishing services aimed at the tourist market may prohibit development in this area, unless special incentives are given by the government, and foreign investors are prepared to invest in the development of the local health facilities.

The issue really is whether complementary polices can be devised and implemented which ensure that access for the poor is not jeopardized. For instance, countries have experimented with dual health care systems (public and private) and with vouchers which could, for instance, be financed by a tax on earnings from "exports" of health services. Equally, exports from a greater inflow of health tourists through the entry of FDI and foreign specialists could generate more opportunities locally which in turn could reduce emigration of skilled personnel especially if the skills of foreign and domestic personnel are complementary which immigration policy can ensure.

There may also be opportunities to provide greater balance through the contracting of private services on behalf of the population, but many of these more highly specialized or esoteric surgeries are limited in the public domain by the simple absence of it, and mechanisms for controlling the introduction of technology (and replication of expensive resources in the private sector to the detriment of quality and sustainability) are not yet in place. Work on national health insurance would also be a key instrument in ensuring equity and re-balancing distribution of financial resources for health and the imp act of health tourism would need to be included in the modelling.

Trade Negotiations in Health Tourism Services

The General Agreement on Trade in Services (GATS) is the first multilateral agreement to provide a framework for regulating trade in services with principles similar to those for trade in goods. Health services include both general and specialized services of medical doctors; deliveries and related services; nursing services; physiotherapeutic and paramedical services; all hospital services; ambulance services; residential health facility services; and medical and dental diagnostic services.

The GATS defines trade in health services along four modes of supply, namely:

— pure trade across borders;
— movement of consumers;
— foreign commercial presence; and,
— movement of natural persons.

These four modes of trade can be applied to the health sector. Table 3 illustrates that there are potentially six different forms of trade in health and health-related services.

Movement of Consumers

Health tourism refers to travel to another country specifically to consume health care services. Health care services can be classified into curative and preventive care. Curative care focuses on providing treatment, diagnostic care, or surgical care provided in hospitals, clinics, or private offices by specialists, physicians, nurses, or allied health professionals. Patients undertake purposeful travel to another country to obtain specialized, curative medical services, or obtain emergency medical care while on vacation or travelling. Preventive services include health spas and resorts which offer alternative forms of healing and stress reduction.

Table 3. Specific Modes and Examples of International Trade in Health Services

Forms of Trade	*Modes of Trade in Health Services*
Movement of consumers	Care for foreign patients
	Health profession educational services for foreign students
Movement of providers	Temporary movement of health personnel to provide services abroad
	Short-term health consulting assignments
Foreign commercial presence	Establishment of foreign companies, subsidiaries, or foreign investment for the management or provision of health services
Pure trade across borders	Trade across borders through mail and electronic media; shipment of samples; analysis of information

In 1996, U.S. exports of health services amounted to approximately US$872 million. Patients came from the U.K., Canada, and Mexico. Medical centres, such as the Mayo Clinic and the Massachusetts General Hospital attract significant inflows of patients from abroad. Johns Hopkins Medical Centre had a rapid increase in the number of foreign patients to 7,200 in 1996.

Patients travel to seek health services for a variety of reasons. The most common reason is related to the lack of availability of a service in one's home country, particularly for experimental procedures or highly specialized care requiring advanced technology or trained personnel. Examples include organ transplantation, cancer treatment, and cardiovascular surgery. For instance, patients travel to Cuba to obtain specialized treatment for vitiligo or psoriasis; and India receives patients for organ transplantation.

A second factor contributing to consumption of health care in another country pertains to the cost of health care. If the quality of a particular service is perceived by the patient to be equivalent with that in the home country, patients may be inclined to travel to obtain less expensive care. This may be particularly true for certain procedures that are not covered under health insurance, such as discretionary care (i.e., cosmetic surgery). The uninsured (more than 40 million in the U.S.) may represent a market of individuals which would choose to travel for more affordable health care. In addition to the cost of care, long waiting lists to obtain services (in places like the U.K. and Canada) may prompt patients to travel abroad, and this may be an incentive for seeking good quality health services in the Caribbean. Another factor related to movement of consumers is potential anonymity and confidentiality, particularly for treatment of certain diseases, cosmetic surgery, or drug addiction therapy.

Cultural reasons may be an incentive for persons residing abroad to travel to seek medical care and health professionals with whom they are comfortable. Patients living along borders between countries may avail themselves of medical services abroad on a regular basis. For instance, households living along the Mexico-U.S. border frequently travel back and forth for medical care.

Movement of Natural Persons

The temporary movement of personnel to provide services abroad is a significant mode of trade in health services. Health professionals migrate to seek improved living and working conditions, and higher pay, often shifting from the public to the private sector. Health professionals may also feel a need to seek professional experience and qualifications elsewhere. The movement of health professionals can temporarily remove shortages in receiving countries, and remittances have a positive effect on countries of origin.

However, developing countries supply 56% of all migrating physicians, but receive less than 11%. While permanent immigration of health professionals can be detrimental to a country, by resulting in a "brain drain," temporary movement provides an opportunity for professionals to upgrade their skills.

The Caribbean is a major supplier of the world's nurses, and approximately 6% of all foreign-trained nurses entering the U.S. are from the Caribbean. Jamaica accounts for the greatest share of nurses from the Region. This has resulted in shortages of experienced nursing staff in the country. To rectify the outflows of nurses, Jamaica currently imports them from Myanmar, Nigeria, and Ghana.

CARICOM encourages the free movement of health professionals throughout the Region, and there is considerable movement of nurses within the Caribbean. In the early 1990s, the Regional Nursing Body established a regional exam that allows nurses to work anywhere in the CARICOM countries. The Nursing Body promotes a common curriculum and regional standards. One of the goals of the Regional Nursing Examination is to stem the rising trend of temporary emigration of nurses from the Region.

A recent survey showed that for 18 months between 1998 and 2000, 170 nurses (33.5%) remained in the Region, 206 nurses (40.7%) emigrated to the U.K., and approximately 130 nurses (25.8%) went to North America. The study estimated that the Caribbean subsidized recipient countries for training of nurses in the amount of $14 million (PAHO/CPC, personal communication).

This assessment was thought to show the positive impact of the regional exam vis-a-vis retaining nurses within the region and promoting movement among Caribbean countries. However, another researcher attributes the slowing of migration to the lack of jobs in North America and other parts of the Caribbean.

The Caribbean Association of Medical Councils (CAMC) is attempting to promote freer movement of physicians throughout the Region by developing a regional examination, promoting registration, licensing, and standards. Presently, all non-University of the West Indies (UWI) graduates interested to work in the Caribbean must take the exam. By 2004, it is expected that all medical graduates will be required to take the examination. While one benefit of this examination is a standardization of medical qualifications within the Region, Medical Boards in the each country will continue to have discretion over who is allowed to practice. This discretionary power has implications for free trade within the Caribbean.

Direct Foreign Investment

There are several benefits to direct foreign investment in the health sector. Opening markets to domestic and foreign competition may contribute to cost reductions in health care, as well as improve the quality of care and range of services provided. However, these results can only occur in an environment where the public and private sectors work together, with the public sector being an effective regulator of the private sector. This is a potential area of weakness for the Caribbean, in that the Ministry of Health is often not involved in decision-making regarding licensing and entry of foreign interests into the health sector.

Some of the barriers to trade relating to foreign direct investment include ownership regulations and economic need limitations. In addition, limits on foreign equity participation can have an effect on the openness of markets to foreign investment.

Cross-border Supply

Cross-border supply refers to the traditional mode of trade between countries. With respect to health services, this includes transfer of information, claims processing, diagnostic services, and telemedicine. The World Health Organization recently noted the increasing importance of cross-border trade in health services, particularly related to sharing of medical information via internet technology. Telemedicine is the practice of medical care using audio, visual, and data communications.

Telemedicine can be used to provide services that are not available locally, such as radiography. In addition, telemedicine can be used to treat patients with chronic disease as part of a more cost-effective, home-based health care strategy. Further, telemedicine can facilitate a second opinion on medical diagnoses and treatment, as well as perform a vital link in the transport and referral of patients from one setting to another. Finally, telemedicine can be used as a training tool to maintain and upgrade the skills of professionals who may not have access to the latest medical information.

Currently, there are few companies that provide travellers with telemedicine facilities. One example is WorldCare International Limited, which began in 1992, and which has affiliates in Asia, Latin America, and the Middle East. This system links travellers to a quality network of highly specialized medical expertise in major medical centres in the U.S.

Some of the potential barriers to trade with respect to telemedicine services include ethical and legal considerations of providing care at a distance, as well as licensure issues for cross-border trade. In addition, most insurance companies do not ordinarily cover services provided through a telemedicine consultation.

REFERENCES

Crell, G.A.C., (1994). "Ecotourism and Health Tourism in the Caribbean," *Bulletin of Eastern Caribbean Affairs*, pp. 39-45 .

Frechtling, D.C. (1997). "Current research on health and tourism issues and future directions," in *Tourism and Health: Risks, Research, and Responses*, Clift, S. and Grabowski, P. eds., Pinter, London.

Hope-Price, G. (1994). *Health Tourism*, Prepared for the World Bank, Dover Convention Centre, Barbados, December 15.

Shepard, D.S. and Vargas, V. (1995). *Health Tourism in Barbados: A Preliminary Assessment*, mimeograph, February 16.

Smith, C. and Jenner, P. (1998). "The Senior's Travel Market," in Travel and Tourism Intelligence, *The Economist Intelligence Unit.*

UNCTAD Secretariat, (1998). "International Trade in Health Services: Difficulties and Opportunities for Developing Countries," in UNCTAD-WHO Joint Publication, International Trade in Health Services: A Development Perspective, Geneva, Switzerland.

UNCTAD-WHO Joint Publication, (1998). *International Trade in Health Services: A Development Perspective,* Geneva, Switzerland.

Warner, D.C., (1998). "The Globalization of Medical Care," in UNCTAD-WHO Joint Publication, *International Trade in Health Services: A Development Perspective*, Geneva, Switzerland.

World Bank, (1993). *World Development Report: Investing in Health*, Washington, D.C. 1993.

8

Ethical and Legal Issues in Medical Tourism

There is no universally accepted definition for "medical tourism," but the phrase generally refers to travelling abroad for health care services. Another approach of medical tourism defined as health care distance from home that is affordable, accessible, available, and acceptable. Medical tourism is not emergent or critical care while out of the country, or expatriate care. Articles and broadcasts on medical tourism are appearing in the press and on the airways with increasing frequency and several guide books were recently published by facilitators and coordinators of medical travel and tourist services on behalf of the medical tourist.

Many countries are working to successfully compete in the medical tourism marketplace by advertising variety of medical, surgical and dental services in comfortable modern facilities. Cost and quality are typically the most important factors patients consider in choosing specific destinations for treatment. However, many patients also consider amenities commonly found in resorts and hotels. Medical tourists travel four corners of the world for executive health evaluations, ophthalmologic care, cosmetic dentistry, and surgery These countries have large, modern medical facilities that are staffed by well-trained physicians who perform complex procedures such as minimally invasive / off-pump heart surgery, correction of congenital cardiac abnormalities in children, thoracic organ transplantation, and implantation of mechanical cardiac devices.

India. Despite the long travel time involved, India is a popular destination for medical tourists. It arguably has the lowest cost and highest quality of all medical tourism destinations and English is widely spoken. Several hospitals are accredited by the Joint Commission International (JCI) and staffed by highly trained physicians. Prices can be obtained in advance and many hospitals bundle services into a package deal that includes the medical procedure and the cost of treating any complications. Hotel accommodations are extra, but hospitals often have hotel rooms or can offer discounts for hotels nearby.

Thailand: This popular destination for medical tourists rivals India in price and quality. Thailand's large tourist industry is one reason it has a better infrastructure and less noticeable poverty than India. Prices are typically not as low as in India, and Thai hospitals do not offer fixed pricing. However, food and lodging during recuperation will likely be less expensive than in India due to Thailand's competitive recreational industry. Bangkok's Bumrungrad International Hospital is a world-class private health care facility built for wealthy Thais, but foreigners comprise more than one-third of its patients.

Singapore: English is also widely spoken in this former British colony, located approximately 1,000 miles south of Bangkok. Singapore has modern, high-quality hospitals and is home to three hospitals accredited by the JCI. Prices are higher than in Thailand or India but are much lower than in the United States.

Central and South America: Mexico has been popular for some time with American patients seeking primary and dental care. But to attract cash-paying American patients for surgical services, health care systems are building hospitals and clinics with the high level of service and amenities that American patients have come to expect. For instance, Americans expect professional medical staff and upscale private rooms in clean, modern facilities. They also expect hightech equipment that American hospitals would possess.

Other Latin American countries provide services as well: For example, Costa Rica is best known for quality dental work, with prices one-third to one-half of those in the United States. Colombia is a favourite destination for cosmetic surgery. Argentina and Brazil have long been known for cut-rate plastic surgery, and more advanced treatments are becoming available. Plenitas is a Buenos Aires-based boutique clinic that arranges medical travel. Although most of the services provided are cosmetic surgeries, it also offers in vitro fertilization and bariatric (weight loss) surgery. Nine Brazilian organizations have established a health care consortium to market Brazil as a medical tourism destination in various countries.

Europe: Northern and Western Europeans have numerous opportunities to get lower-cost medical and dental care. Germans favour Szczecin, Poland, less than 100 miles from Berlin, for low-cost, high-quality dental work. Sopron, Hungary, less than an hour's drive from Vienna, Austria, caters to medical tourists. Sopron has more than 200 dentists and 200 optometrists, 10 times as many as would be expected in a town of 20,000 people.

South Africa: has been very successful selling medical services combined with tourism activities such as Safaris.

For some countries, the rationale for engaging in medical tourism is to improve their Gross Domestic Product (GDP) as overseas patients bring needed cash for procedures. GDP is the primary indicator used to gauge the health of country's economy. It represents the total dollar value of all goods and services produced over a specific time period. Another commonly cited reason for growth of foreign medical sites is a belief that overseas patients expect an even higher standard of care than had been typical their home country, thus promoting hospitals to upgrade their institutions as to remain competitive in a thriving market. India has a reputation for high quality care in a number of major hospitals; has the important advantage of lower cost than most other destinations, at approximately 10 percent Gross Domestic Product (GDP) of the cost of U.S. The cost savings associated with growth of foreign medical sites cannot be overstated. While the costs vary geographically, the average surgical procedure performed in Asia will cost only 20% to 25% as much as the comparable American procedure.

Health care might seem the most, local rooted form of practices, medical interventions and are moving to offshore regions where treatment is more affordable that the U.S. for many reason:

— *Labour Costs.* In the United States, labour costs equal more than half of hospital operating revenue, on the average.. Wage rates and other labour costs are lower overseas; specifics were not available, but as one example, at Fortis hospitals in India

  - Doctors earn about 40 percent less than comparable physicians in the United States.
  - Median nurses' salaries are one-fifth to one-twentieth of those in the United States.
  - The wages of unskilled and semiskilled labour, such as janitors and orderlies, are also much less.
  - These lower labour costs make it much less expensive to build and operate hospitals in other countries.
- *Less (or No) Third-Party Payment*: Markets tend to be bureaucratic and stifling when insurers or governments pay most medical bills. In the United States, third parties (insurers, employers and government) pay for about 87 percent of health care. So patients spend only 13 cents out of pocket for every dollar they spend on their health care. As a result, they do not shop like consumers do when they are spending their own money, and the providers who serve them rarely compete for their business based on price.
- *Price Transparency and Package Pricing*: One criticism of American hospitals and clinics is that prices are difficult to obtain and often meaningless when they are disclosed. Patients who ask potential providers to quote a price are likely to be disappointed. In fact, many people have little idea of the cost of medical treatments. A recent Harris Poll found:
  - Consumers can guess the price of a new Honda Accord within $1,000, but when asked to estimate the cost of a four-day hospital stay; those same consumers were off by $12,000
  - Furthermore, 68 percent of those who had received recent medical care did not know the cost until the bill arrived, and 11 percent said they never learned the cost at all.

In the international health care marketplace, the situation is quite different. Package prices are common, and medical travel intermediaries help patients compare prices. Even providers who do not offer fixed pricing will provide reasonably accurate price quotes. As a result, medical centres and clinics that treat large numbers of medical tourists routinely quote prices in advance and look for ways to reduce patients' costs.

— *Few Cross-Subsidies*: In American full-service non-profit general hospitals, revenues from treatments for some patients are used to cover the costs of providing treatments to other patients. This cross-subsidisation is possible because some medical procedures produce more revenue than it costs to provide them. For example, the revenue from routine heart catheterization procedures or diagnostic imaging systems in a community hospital might be used to subsidize indigent health care or the cost of operating the emergency room. Thismeansthata hospital's charges for the heart procedure m ore than cover its costs, but its charges for emergency room care do not cover those costs. If there is no competition for the business of heart patients in the hospital's service area, it can cross-subsidize without losing revenue. However, a provider who does not cross-subsidize could offer the cardiac treatment for a lower price or could make a profit charging the same price. In the United States, such providers have emerged in the form of highly efficient specialty hospitals. Non-profit community hospitals complain that specialty hospitals skim off lucrative surgeries but do not provide the services that community hospitals do, such as emergency departments and charity care for the uninsured. This has led to a moratorium on new specialty hospitals in the Medicare program.

— *Streamlined Services*: Some foreign medical providers operate highly efficient "focused factories." These are specialty clinics and hospitals where tasks and procedures have been streamlined for the highest efficiency, similar to the way an automotive plant operates. For example, Fortis Healthcare's Rajan Dhall Hospital in New Delhi uses a business model that combines the personalized service of the hotel industry with the industrial processes of an automaker; both industries in which its senior executives have experience. Jasbir Grewal, Rajan Dhall's vice president for operations, spent years working forawell-known hotel chain. He describes their hospital as "a hotel providing clinical medical excellence." Fortis chairman Harpal Singh, who cam e from the automotive industry, emphasizes the need to streamline processes in such a way that procedures can be performed quickly and efficiently.

— *Limited Malpractice Liability*: Malpractice litigation costs are also lower in other countries than in the United States. In addition, one of the most significant differences in health care cost between the U.S. and global competitors stem from malpractice insurance premiums. In Thailand, for example, the average doctor will pay approximately $5,000 in medical malpractice insurance for one year's coverage. Contrast this with malpractice premiums in the U.S., which can cost up to $100,000 a year for specialist, and a major source of Thailand's savings become clear. Thailand does not compensate victims of negligence for noneconomic damages, and malpractice awards are far lower than in the United States. As the data indicates, the difference in cost to the consumer is even greater than the savings experienced by insurance companies, assuming the medical cost in the U.S. continue to trend upward.

— *Fewer Regulations*: Excessive health care regulations in the United States prevent American hospitals from making the sort of collaborative arrangements many international hospitals use. For instance, facilities abroad can structure physicians' compensation to create financial incentives for the doctors to provide efficient care, whereas American hospitals usually cannot. The reason is physician compensation arrangements in American hospitals cannot violate the Stark (anti-kickback) laws. Foreign hospitals can also employ physicians directly; a practice prohibited by many states. For instance, physicians in India contract with hospitals to provide a certain number of hours per month in return for a guaranteed fixed fee. Patients select the hospital based on reputation and then choose an appropriate doctor who works with the hospital. In this regard, physicians depend on hospitals for business rather than the other way around.

The significant cost savings available oversea means little, however, unless it motivates persons to go through the hassle and risk of travel before and after surgery and recovering in foreign environment. A study by Deloitte in 2009, suggests that eight percent indicated that they sought health care services outside their immediate community; over forty percent say they would travel outside their immediate area if their physician recommended it or for a fifty percent cost savings. In 2008, fewer consumers reported going to a distant hospital; one percent reported using an offshore health care provider. The larger number of person willing to travel to abroad for discount surgical procedures highlights the importance of financial incentives in the growth of foreign medical sites and the potential impact of outsourcing of health care could have upon the U.S. health care system in the future.

Quality and Safety in Medical Tourism

The critical challenge for potential medical tourists is to select the best possible destination for the specific services needed. Although medical tourism offers benefit for many patients, quality of care issues abound. Many hospitals that advertise heavily to medical tourists are located in low-cost, developing countries that may experiencing social, political, and cultural problems. These issues may detract from quality of care received, thus resulting in a less than optimal environment for the medical tourist seeking quality health care. There are also concerns regarding lengthy airplane trips needed to travel to distant countries. These long trips have been associated with known health risks, such as lung disease and thrombosis. The lower oxygen levels on airplanes in flight could become problematic for patients with lung disease taking a flight to a developing country, sometimes in excess of 14 hours. Long flights can also contribute to development of deep vein thrombosis (DVT). Both of these conditions are of serious concern for surgical patients. Other quality issues include complications that might result from vacation activities and travel in the postoperative periods and follow-up care, as well as adequate communication between provider and patients. Provisions to assure the quality of long-term, follow-up care, and provide for the cost of the care need to be considered to before undergoing procedures in another country. Additionally, cultural barriers and language, including medical jargon, may be problematic, even with the assistance of interpreters. Serious misunderstanding may occur on both the part of the patient and the provider. Both the patient and provider need to share with each other all necessary information before initiating the procedure designed to promote quality outcomes.

Another issue is the quality of the foreign hospital environment. Patient should carefully assess the quality and standard that they expect and have been promised. This assessment should include the environment outside the hospital. In some countries the quality of the water, as well as hygienic standard, m ay vary from patients' expectations and may compromise thei. convalescence. For instance, the World Health Organization (2008) reported that data collected in 2006 from 132 countries demonstrated that 31 countries (or 23.5%) have less 100 percent screening for at least four common infection markers: HIV, HBV, HCV, and syphilis. WHO noted that many countries cannot provide complete information related to the screening process, even when testing of blood products; the testing may often be incomplete or lack of a quality assurance mechanism. Thus, patients risk becoming sicker through their travel to another country, rather than gaining an improved state of health. While the number of foreign medical sites continues to increase, issues remain about how to best monitor quality and patient safety.

Measuring Quality

Despite claims of high U.S. standards, results vary widely by hospital. Consider one of the most commonly performed procedures in the United States today, coronary artery bypass graft (CABG) surgery:

— Hospitals in California that perform CABG surgery have an average mortality rate of nearly 3 percent (2.91).

— The California average is nearly four times higher than the Cleveland Clinic, considered the best hospital in the nation by *U.S. News & World Report.*

Closer inspection of California hospitals shows wide variations in quality:

— The University of California Davis Medical Centre experienced no deaths among the 136 patients receiving CABG surgery in 2003.

— Fountain Valley's mortality rate of 2.14 percent was below the state average of 2.91 percent.

— Desert Regional Medical Centre, which performed a similar volume of surgeries, had a mortality rate of more than 6 percent, twice the California average and 10 times Cleveland Clinic's average.

— Beverly Hospital performs few CABG procedures, which may explain its high mortality rate of 13.79 percent.

How does the quality of facilities overseas compare to those in the United States? Some of the more prestigious providers, such as Apollo Hospital Group and Wockhardt Hospitals (which is affiliated with Harvard Medical School) in India, and Bumrungrad International Hospital in Thailand, offer a better level of care than the average community hospital in the U.S.

In comparison, Bumrungrad International Hospital in Bangkok, Thailand, is a modern multi-speciality hospital with 554 beds, accredited by the Joint Commission International. Its main 12-story building was constructed in 1997 to comply with U.S. hospital building and safety standards. The medical staff of more than 900 includes about 200 U.S. board-certified physicians. Many others hold licenses in Australia, Europe and Japan. A team of 800 nurses assists with patient care.

Bumrungrad tracks more than 500 measures of quality and patient safety. It treats about 430,000 medical tourists a year from 190 different countries. This number included nearly 60,000 American patients in 2005. Bumrungrad is equipped with all the latest diagnostic equipment. It has 150 clinical exam suites, two cardiac catheterization labs and 19 operating theatres, two of which are specifically designed for cardiac surgeries.

The hospital uses Global Care Solutions' Hospital 2000®, a sophisticated health information technology system. This software is designed to recognize and prevent dangerous drug interactions, store patient records electronically and fully integrate all areas of patient management and hospital operations. The hospital staff assists patients with travel arrangements, airport pickup, interpreters and lodging if needed. Seventy-five percent of Bumrungrad's patients pay cash for services.

As in the U.S., many hospitals abroad do not disclose recognized quality indicators. But most hospitals that compete on the international level generally do, such as:

— Dartmouth Hitchcock Medical Centre in New Hampshire and Ohio's Cleveland Clinic have quality indicators on their Web sites.

- — National University Hospital Singapore also discloses information demonstrating that its quality compares very favourably internationally.
- — India's Apollo Hospital Group has devised a clinical excellence model to ensure its quality meets international health care standards across all its hospital.
- — Other Indian hospitals are working to create standards for reporting performance measures.

Electronic Medical Records

Because potential medical tourists must first be evaluated remotely, most large health care providers and medical intermediaries for patients use electronic medical records (EMRs) to store and access patient files. Patients can then discuss the procedures with potential physicians via conference call. Modern hospitals abroad also use information technology to identify potential drug interactions, manage patient caseloads and store radiology and laboratory test results.

By contrast, only about one out of four U.S. hospitals store medical records electronically. Third parties pay 87 percent of medical bills in the U.S. health care system, and most of the third parties do not reimburse physicians or hospitals for the use of EMRs. Since others pay the bills, patients usually do not choose hospitals or physicians based on their use of EMRs.

Hospital Accreditation

How does the quality of facilities overseas compare to those in the U.S? The Joint Commission International (JCI), a subsidiary of the U.S. Joint Commission is the health care industry's official accreditation institution, in addition to providing educational and consulting services to hospitals around the world. It has increased the number of approved foreign medical sites from 76 in 2005 to over 220 in 2008 12. Both JCI and the International Organization of Standardization (ISO) are able to provide useful and reassuring benchmarks for patients in selecting offshore medical facilities. In lieu of the JCI, some countries are adopting their own accreditation standards. For instance, the Indian Healthcare Federation is developing accreditation standards for its members in an attempt to reassure potential patients about India's high quality health care.

Hospital Affiliation

Some foreign hospitals are owned, managed or affiliated with prestigious American universities or health care systems:

- The Cleveland Clinic owns facilities in Canada and Vienna, Austria; and in Abu Dhabi, the clinic already manages an existing facility and is building a new hospital.
- Wockhardt (India) is affiliated with Harvard Medical School.
- Hospital Punta Pacifica in Panama City, Panama, is an affiliate of U.S.-based Johns Hopkins International.
- JCI-accredited International Medical Centre in Singapore is also affiliated with Johns Hopkins International.
- Dallas-based International Hospital Corp. is building and operating hospitals in Mexico that meet American standards.
- Bumrungrad International Hospital in Thailand has an American management team to provide American-style care.

Physician Credentials

Foreign health care providers and medical travel intermediaries also compete on quality by touting the credentials of the medical staff. These physicians are often U.S. board-certified, while others have internationally respected credentials. Many of the physicians working with medical tourists were trained in the United States, Australia, Canada or Europe. Nearly two-thirds of the physicians who work with Planet Hospital have either fellowship with medical societies in the United States or the United Kingdom, or are certified for a particular specialty by a medical board.

Online Communities

Potential patients can get some idea of the safety and quality of medical providers by searching online for testimonies of patients who have had surgery abroad. These Internet communities facilitate the exchange of information about providers, including facility cleanliness, convenience, price, satisfaction with medical services and the availability of lodging while recuperating. Professional websites are also helpful in identifying quality care. The International Society of Plastic surgery certifies approximately 1,500 surgeons in 73 countries who meet U.S. standards of care. The American Dental Association website includes information addressing travel, dental care, and dental tourism. This site provided a link to A Traveller's Guide to Denta Care, which is available through Global Dental Safety and Asepsis Procedures The American Medical Association (AMA) has developed guiding principles for employers, insurance companies, and other bodies that facilitate or offer incentives for care outside the U.S. These principles were adopted at the June 17, 2008, annual session of the AMA. The principles stipulate the following:

— international care must be voluntary and provided by accredited institutions
— financial incentives should not limit or restrict patient options inappropriately
— continuity of care, including coverage of costs upon return, should be provided
— patients should be informed of their rights and legal recourse before travel
— patients should have access to licensing, outcome, and accrediting information when seeking care
— medical record transfers should comply with the Health Insurance Portability and Accountability Act guidelines
— patients should be informed of the potential risks of combining surgical procedures with long flights and vacation activities.

PlasticSurgeryJourneys.com has built such a community. Members, including both former and prospective patients, can exchange information in online discussion forums on such topics as destinations, specific physicians and types of surgery. Members answer questions about side effects, complications and occasionally even discuss patients who have died from surgery. A few members who had cosmetic surgery have even posted before-and-after photos. If a facility performed low-quality work on a member, others in the community know to avoid the provider. For example, patients who were disfigured by Mexican cosmetic surgeons created a Web site to warn would-be patients. HealthMedicalTourism.org is another website with a forum where members can interact.

Risks and Adverse Outcomes

All surgical procedures carry an accessory amount of risk; even with the most skilled physicians, patients may have adverse outcomes. When a medical tourist experiences injury or even death, it is natural to wonder whether a poorly trained physician or substandard hospital played a part. Of course, sometimes adverse events are due to the patient's preexisting health conditions or other factors not the fault of the physician; but, as with any service providers, doctors aren't perfect.

Actor Steve McQueen is one of the most recognizable "medical tourists" to travel abroad for treatment with laetrile. Laetrile is a compound that contains a chemical called amygdalin, is found in the pits of many fruits, raw nuts, and plants. It is believed that the active anticancer ingredient in laetrile is cyanide. Laetrile is given by mouth as a pill or by intravenous injection. Laetrile has shown little anticancer effect in laboratory studies, animal studies, or human studies. The side effects are like the symptoms of cyanide poisoning. Laetrile is not approved by the US Food and Drug Administration (FDA). McQueen suffered from mesothelioma, an incurable cancer of the lungs related to asbestos exposure, and in 1980 he travelled to Mexico for laetrile treatment. McQueen initially reported success from the treatment, but he eventually died in November of 1980 after surgery to remove a cancerous mass from his body. Although McQueen did not survive and the effectiveness of laetrile is widely criticized by the medical community, because of lack of opportunity to try the lateral treatment in the U.S. and which may spur cancer patients and others to travel abroad for medical treatment.

In addition, Joshua Goldberg's death at Bumrungrad International provides a sobering account of the risks of medical tourism. Bumrungrad International Hospital admitted Josh Goldberg on February 12, 2006 after he complained of an "abrasion on his left leg that resulted in pain, swelling, and loss of feeling and motion. Allegedly, Mr. Goldberg died twelve days later on February 24 after being administered a cocktail of twenty drugs, six of which were contraindicated." Mr. Goldberg's family contends that the hospital made no resuscitation attempt after discovering Mr. Goldberg's body, and a report of an independent medical examiner hired by the deceased's family supports their allegation. Mr. Goldberg's death remains the subject of litigation both domestically and abroad. His alleged experience casts a dark pall over medical standards abroad.

Little evidence exists to indicate that botched operations are a widespread problem in the medical tourism industry. Anecdotal evidence tends to involve cosmetic surgery patients who went to facilities that were not screened by a respected intermediary or whose physicians' credentials were not checked. Sometimes complications from cosmetic surgery are due to a patient's having too many procedures performed too soon. Most American physicians advise against multiple or consecutive cosmetic surgeries in a short period of time. But patients often have limited time off from work and consider travel and recuperative time as part of the cost of surgery. Thus they are tempted to economize by having more work done than is medically recommended.

Some foreign physicians entice patients with package deals that combine multiple surgeries for one low price. It is not uncommon for South American doctors to offer package prices that include full body liposuction, a breast lift or augmentation (with implant) and a tummy tuck. The package price can be as low as $6,500 (plus travel and lodging) in Colombia, Costa Rica or Mexico. The comparable surgery costs $12,000 to $15,000 and sometimes as much as $30,000 in the U.S.. Women who receive that much cosmetic surgery at one time often find recuperation slow and extremely painful. They may also need postoperative monitoring in a clinic for several days with intravenous antibiotics and blood transfusions, all of which can add several thousand dollars to their overall cost.

The "Web-based intermediaries mentioned elsewhere in this study could help potential patients more carefully choose a destination and physician through a rating system similar to those found for travel and hotels on eBay, Orbitz, Travelocity or Expedia." A rating system would help steer patients to facilities that have more satisfied customers. Health care providers that fail to supply the quality and level of service American patients expect would be blackballed, or at the very least learn valuable lessons about what patients want.

Foreign laws governing medical liability are not as strict as those in the U.S., nor are malpractice compensation awards as generous. Foreign physicians typically do not carry the same level of malpractice insurance as physicians practicing in the U.S. The threshold for malpractice is higher outside the United States, and there is limited recourse through the court system in some countries. Injured patients may not even have the right to sue at all.

Moreover, a medical tourist would have no recourse through the American court system. It is doubtful an American court would hold an intermediary liable since medical tourism "matchmakers" are not health care providers, and, thus cannot commit malpractice. Reputable facilities abroad will work hard to prevent and correct problems. Although it rarely happens, patients may have to travel back for follow-up care if they do not have a U.S. physician willing to provide it. A patient may travel overseas again because the cost of treating unexpected complications is lower abroad. Additionally, some providers include treatment for complications in their package price.

Furthermore, there are offshore insurance companies offering medical malpractice insurance by contract. Medical tourists who have little recourse in foreign courts when malpractice occurs have another option: they can purchase a medical malpractice policy that pays in the event a procedure is botched from AOS Assurance Company Limited, an insurer based in Barbados. One of the ways AOS ensures quality (and reduces its risk) is by covering only procedures performed in accredited hospitals by credentialed physicians. For instance, "an American patient needing angioplasty can obtain $250,000 of coverage for a fee of $1,124.55. A patient wanting $100,000 in financial protection against a botched face-lift would pay $225." In the event of medical malpractice, AOS Assurance Company Limited will compensate insured patients or their beneficiaries for lost wages, repair costs, out-of-pocket expenses, rehabilitation, severe disfigurement, loss of reproductive capacity and death. Claims are administered by an independent, Canadian-based firm, Crawford & Company.

Apart from patient safety, but another safety concern, is how medical waste is handled at foreign medical sites. Simply defined, medical waste includes used needles, soiled dressings, blood, body parts, chemical, pharmaceuticals, expired medicines, scalpels, medical devices, and radioactive materials. According to World Health Organization (WHO), approximately twenty percent of the wasted generated from health care facilities is hazardous. Hazardous materials could be infectious, toxic, or radioactive. Medical waste is a serious concern in the third world especially, in countries with little or no enforcement on medical hazardous materials. According to the author; in Costa Rica, hospitals in San Jose produce 17 tons of waste a day and about twenty five percent of it is classified as biohazardous. These materials are disposed of in bright red plastic bags. The contents pose a health and safety risk to scavengers who comb landfills to gather items for recycling or financial rewards. One might argue that the medical accreditation process may help with medical waste concerns. The challenge is large, since medical accreditation considers the patient and foremost, much akin the way traditional tourism caters to tourist.

Ethical and Legal Considerations

It appears that medical tourism in our global economy is here to stay. One obvious concern is the ethical and legal uncertainty regarding medical tourism. What rights do patients have? There is no current international legal regulation of medical tourism. However, there are many agencies that provide services to potential patients who want foreign medical and surgical health care. These agencies help patients select a country, facility, and provider. They determine prices and collect payments, assemble and transit medical records, and arrange travel and accommodations. Additionally, they may arrange for postoperative follow-up in the patient's own community after they return. For example is MedRetreat, a U.S. based medical tourism service agent facilitating health care needs and travel for desire of Americans. MedRetreat created a network of pre-qualified hospitals from which a client can choose. For medical tourists who may want to file malpractice claims in the U.S., medical tourism firms make attractive defendants because they are not encumbered with personal jurisdiction problems that might protect negligent foreign physicians. A firm that is incorporated in or has its principal place of business in a particular state is always subject to that state's jurisdiction. Consequently, medical-tourism plaintiffs might try to hold the medical-tourism firms they used liable for including foreign providers who were negligent on their network. Plaintiffs could invoke a number of theories to hold medical-tourism firms liable, including corporate negligence, the informed consent doctrine, and vicarious liability. However, none of these theories fit perfectly in the medical tourism context.

What rights do plans administrators have to outsource medical, surgical, or hospital care benefits overseas? Given the broad scope of the Employee Retirement Income Security Act of 1974 (ERISA). The act provides, in relevant part as follows:

- A health insurance carrier, health maintenance organization, or other managed care entity for a health care plan has duty to exercise ordinary care when making health care treatment decisions and is liable for damages for harm to an insured or enrollee proximate caused by its failure to exercise such ordinary care.
- A health insurance carrier, health maintenance organization, or other managed care entity for a health care plan is also liable for damages for harm to an insured or enrollee proximately caused by the health care decisions made by:
  - employees,
  - agents,
  - ostensible agents, or
  - representative who are acting on its behalf and over whom it has the right to exercise influence or control or has actually exercised influence or control which result in the failure to exercise ordinary care.

ERISA reflects the government's belief that employee benefit and welfare plans play such an important role in interstate commerce that these plans represent a national public interest. Therefore, ERISA seeks to ensure the sound management and application of employee benefit and welfare plans in the U.S. What roles do World Trade

Organization (WTO) and World Health Organization (WHO) play in globalization of health care? WTO helps member nations attain fair trade of outsourcing of medical services and WHO helps member nations attain highest possible levels of health. Every country has different standards, rules and regulations that have restrained a wider use of cross border delivery and seeking of medical care. The WTO played a pivotal role in mediating internally agreed upon rules and settling disputes among country as far as trade in health good and services is concerned. The WTO played in the arena of public health to make pharmaceutical products more accessible to low and middle income countries and provides a description of possible consequences for one such policy that was meant to provide flexibility for trade in drugs. Although prohibitively high drug prices is the primary barrier to affordable medicines for developing nations, even the developed nations have started facing their own problems with respect to access to affordable care, more in the form of services. U.S. has seen rising numbers of individuals who either do not have health insurance or have insurance or are routinely denied catastrophically expensive care. Rising costs of medical care has fostered cross-border outsource of health care services and international medical tourism has become a viable alternative for health care providers and potential patients.

With the North American Free Trade Agreement (NAFTA), the health care sectors of the United States, Canada, and Mexico are becoming more economically integrated. NAFTA poses major challenges to the realization of the international human rights. These include:

— Cross Border Trade in Medical Products,
— Cross Border Trade in Medical Services, and the attendant investment protections,
— Portability and Comparability of Health Insurance Coverage, and
— Protection of Public Health Insurance Programs.

The United States, Mexico, and Canada all provide public health insurance programs either to the entire population as in Canada or to vulnerable groups as in the United States. None of these countries have private, for-profit providers and insurers able to provide universal and affordable health coverage and care in a truly free market. Private insurers and for-profit providers should not profit from the care of the healthy and wealthy in ways that compromise the public programs that serve the poor and seriously ill. Nor should they be allowed to use NAFTA processes to compromise public programs.

For the United States, globalization of health care encompasses both exporting patients (medical tourism) and importing medical services (outsourcing). This medical trade has the potential to increase competition and efficiency in the United States. Princeton University health economist Uwe Reinhardt says the effect of global competition on American health care could rival the impact of Japanese automakers on the U.S. auto industry forcing domestic producers to improve quality and to offer consumers more choices.

Apart from patient travel, many medical tasks can be outsourced to skilled professionals abroad when the physical presence of a physician is unnecessary. This can include long distance collaboration incorporating the services of foreign medical staff into the practices of American medical providers. Global competitors can build facilities closer to the United States and selectively contract with U.S. health insurers.

Outsourcing Medical Services

Information technology makes it possible to provide many medical services remotely, including outsourcing them to other countries. Telemedicine the use of information technology to treat or monitor patients remotely by telephone, Webcam or video feed is becoming common in areas where physicians are scarce. It gives rural residents access to specialists and will probably become the preferred way to monitor patients with chronic conditions. Outsourcing often results in lower costs, higher quality and greater convenience. Some clerical tasks, such as medical transcription entering physician notes and dictation into a patient's electronic medical record are already outsourced. American hospitals increasingly use radiologists in India and other countries to read X-rays. For instance, Night Hawk Radiology Services contracts with American board-certified physicians living in Australia for overnight interpretations of X-rays and scans. Other medical tasks that don't require the physical presence of a physician could also be outsourced to lower-cost doctors abroad. The British National Health Service (NHS) is considering using doctors in India to read some lab tests and MRI scans. Planet Hospital has offered to work with U.S. hospitals to set up local imaging centres that would use physicians in India to read imaging scans. An MRI scan could be performed profitably for as little as $400 to $500, far less than typical U.S. prices.

Opportunities for Collaboration

Helping patients properly manage a chronic condition is often complex and time consuming. Outcomes could be improved if teams of medical providers worked together to improve all aspects of medical treatment through aggressive case management. When multiple physicians are treating a patient, a case manager could ensure that all physicians are coordinating their efforts. However, such close monitoring and interaction is labour-intensive and costly. Often these tasks are not reimbursed or are reimbursed at rates lower than the cost of providing them. A potential solution is for American health care providers to collaborate with low-cost providers in developing countries by having them perform these labour-intensive tasks that don't require the physical presence of a physician.

Telemedicine, which involves remote consultation, monitoring and treatment of patients, is increasingly being used in disease management programs. Past research has already shown that telemedicine can improve adherence to protocols and increase convenience for patients with chronic ailments. Thus, it is a logical to outsource some of disease management or remote health coaching to places where labour costs are lower.

Creating New Heath Insurance Plans

Currently, most insurers do not include foreign providers in their networks, but they may in the future. Mercer Health, an employee benefits consulting firm, is working with several Fortune 500 employers to take advantage of medical travel. Several health insurers are also experimenting with international coverage. Milica Bookman, a professor at St. Joseph University, predicts that by 2009, it will become increasingly common for mainstream health insurers to include foreign providers in their networks. The simple answer is that no one knows how the global competition will affect medical tourism in 2009 and beyond. The following are some examples of insurance products that already use foreign providers.

Access Baja

BlueShield of California has a health network designed for people who choose to get their medical care in Mexico. Access Baja was implemented a year after California passed legislation in 1999 allowing the state's insurers to reimburse providers in Mexico. Although many of the enrollees are Mexican nationals who cross the U.S. border each day to work, employers on both sides of the border can offer this plan to their workers. However, the plan requires enrollees to live within 50 miles of the border to easily access the Mexican primary care physicians in the BlueShield network. By 2005, nearly 40,000 people had signed up for coverage offered by Mexican health care providers. Because Mexican medical care costs less, Access Baja premiums are less than two-thirds the cost of the alternative BlueShield of California plans. Hispanic enrollees can have a doctor who is fluent in Spanish and understands their culture. An added convenience is that Mexican physicians are often available for same-day appointments, as well as evenings and on weekends.

Networks with Foreign Hospitals

Some health plans take advantage of the potential in allowing enrollees to travel abroad for lower-cost treatments. In February 2007, BlueCross BlueShield of South Carolina added Bumrungrad International Hospital in Thailand to its network. South Carolina BlueCross BlueShield does not plan to require patients to go abroad for lower-cost care, nor is it actively considering using financial incentives to encourage patients to travel abroad. Rather it is a value-added service available to members who request it. While no patients have thus far taken advantage of this service, it may benefit underinsured patients facing steep out-of-pocket payments.

Other Options

Insurers are hopeful that medical tourism will help to reduce treatment costs and improve margins, while employers are seeking reduced health care costs. It is yet to be determined whether these pilot plans will be adopted on a broad scale and whether employers or patients will receive the benefit of cost savings via reduced premiums, co-payments or deductibles. As the medical tourism trend grows, other U.S.-based companies in the health industry are looking at ways to offer medical travel that is at least partially covered by health insurance.

— Anthem Blue Cross and Blue Shield (WellPoint) located in Wisconsin. Promoting to clients for certain elective procedures. The program will start with Delhi and Bangalore facilities and later expand to all JCI, accredited Apollo Hospitals. Pilot project will cover about 700 group members. All financial details, including travel and medical arrangements, will be managed by Anthem WellPoint United Group Program.

— United Group Program, a third party administrator located in Florida. Promoting medical tourism for elective surgical care to more than 200,000 individuals covered through self-funded health plans and fully insured, mini-med plans in Bumrungrad Thailand.

— Blue Shield and Health Net sell discounted health insurance policies that encourage potential patient to get most of their care in Mexico. This plan covers about 20,000 patients, and focused on employers that hire a large number of Mexican immigrants.

— Blue Cross Blue Shield South Carolina is focusing efforts in Thailand through its subsidiary, Companion Global Health, Inc., that streamlines access to care for members and uninsured at Bumrungrad International Hospital in Bangkok.

Over the next few years, at least 40 company-sponsored health plans will offer overseas options through United Group Programs, a health insurer in Boca Raton, Florida.

In 2006, West Virginia's legislature held hearings on the possibility of including foreign hospitals in its state employees' health plan network. West Virginia HB 2841 Bill introduced Feb. 7, 2007 Program to establish incentives for covered employees who elect to obtain medical care or medical procedures in foreign health care facilities accredited by the Joint Commission International (JCI) Incentives included:

- — Waiver of all co-payments and deductibles payments
- — Payment of round-trip airfare for covered employee and one companion
- — Lodging expenses in the foreign country for the covered employee and companion
- — Payment to the covered employee's hiring agency for seven days of paid sick leave
- — Rebate to covered employee of not more than 20 percent of cost savings The West Virginia 12 HB 2841 Bill died in committee.

Colorado14 07-1143 Bill introduced in 2007. Program to establish incentives for state employees covered under state group benefit plans who elect to obtain medical care in a foreign health care facility where the cost of such care is lower. The Colorado 14 07 -1143 Bill was postponed indefinitely in the House Committee on Business Affairs and Labour. These bills were attempted to provide services for potential patient who wants offshore medical and surgical care.

The medical tourism firms U.S. Health and Planet Hospital are in the process of creating health insurance products that combine American-based primary care with foreign travel for expensive procedures.

Planet Hospital is working with a major insurer to design a low-cost health plan. Initially, Planet Hospital plans to roll out a limited benefit plan, sometimes referred to as a "mini-med" plan, based on the casualty insurance model where the benefit is a specific sum of money. These types of plans generally provide coverage for a limited number of physician visits each year, a limited amount of inpatient care and sometimes coverage for prescription drugs. Mini-med policies typically cap benefits at a maximum of about $25,000 annually. Since the amounts these policies will pay are relatively low, patients can expect significant cost-sharing for medical care. But this provides an incentive for patients to carefully shop to avoid high out-of-pocket costs.

The unique part of Planet Hospital's plan is that it will reimburse patients the same amount for each particular service, regardless of where it is performed. Thus a patient could significantly lower out-of-pocket costs by going abroad for treatment. For instance, an enrollee who needs a heart procedure could easily spend more than $50,000 at a hospital in the United States. A mini-med policy may pay only $10,000 toward the cost. But abroad, the same surgery could cost less than $10,000, including travel, thus making the mini-med a sensible and affordable alternative. Because coverage is limited, this policy will cost about $50 to $100 a month, only a fraction of a traditional health plan.

Planet Hospitals' first step will be a health plan aimed at El Salvadorans living in the United States. Enrollees would receive a limited number of primary care visits locally under the plan and could travel to El Salvador for covered major medical needs. If the plan proves successful, additional ones will follow for countries such as Mexico and India. Coverage under one of these "mini-med" plans might cost a family as little as $200 per month.

Effects of Increased Competition on in Health Care Markets

Global competition could lower the cost of some medical procedures. At the same time, increased international competition for qualified medical personnel could raise labour costs in the United States. If foreign medical students, physicians and nurses currently in America choose to work overseas, there may be shortages of workers in some medical specialities in the United States, and wages for these workers will rise. This is especially likely in areas of medicine not easily outsourced. For example, radiology is relatively easy to outsource since it does not require the radiologist to be physically present. Although radiology has been one of the highest-paid specialities in medicine, that is likely to change in the future since reading X-rays and other scans can easily be outsourced. On the other hand, outsourcing would have little effect on the inherently local practice of emergency room medicine.

Global medical competition could also exacerbate the shortage of primary care physicians in the United States. Today nearly one-quarter of practicing physicians in the United States attended a foreign medical school. Indeed, each year nearly one-quarter of slots in U.S. medical residency programs are filled by foreigners. Greater opportunities in their native countries and in other countries could reduce the number of foreign physicians and nurses practicing in the

United States. It could also encourage more of them to return home after they receive training. Many foreign medical graduates work in underserved rural areas, would be especially hard hit. Also, due to an ongoing nursing shortage, American hospitals recruit foreign nurses to fill vacancies. A smaller supply of foreign physicians and nurses willing to work in the United States could strain the U.S. health care system by raising labour costs.

Today many developing countries, including African and Asia countries are experiencing shortages of physicians and nurses.. Because of the opportunity to earn more in Europe and the United States, many physicians trained in developing countries emigrate for more opportunities to work for higher pay and entrepreneurial opportunities in developed countries. Critics in developing countries claim that health care facilities and providers that serve medical tourists will treat only foreign patients to the exclusion of native-born poor residents. This is unlikely, since most hospitals in developing countries cannot survive on cash-paying medical tourists alone. But even if specific hospitals in developing countries are open only to foreigners and local elites, the health care systems of these countries will be enriched by the influx of revenue, thus would benefit the local population by increasing their access to medical care.

Policy Issues

Health care globalization, including medical tourism and medical outsourcing, has the potential to lower costs and increase competition in the American health care industry. However, there are numerous obstacles to incorporating foreign health care providers into the U.S. health care system. Some of these barriers are the result of entrenched interest groups that do not want to compete with low-cost providers. Federal and state laws also create a number of obstacles to Americans seeking treatment abroad, including outdated laws supposedly intended to protect consumers that now merely increase costs and reduce convenience, for example ERISA may limit incentive, state insurance commissioner, and state licensure laws. Finally, state and federal regulations currently restrict public providers from outsourcing expensive medical procedures, for example Federal STARK laws may inhibit collaboration.

In addition, federal regulations make it difficult for private plans to offer financial rewards to enrollees willing to seek care abroad. This is significant because insurance pays the bills for most U.S. patients and surveys find that patients are unwilling to travel long distances for health care of the same quality they could receive at home unless they have a financial incentive to do so.

State Licensing Laws

Recent advances in information technology allow a radiologist to read X-rays from India just as easily as an American radiologist could read them from a home office. However, the practice of medicine is regulated by state medical boards, which generally require a physician to be licensed in the state where the patient receives treatment. Thus, state licensing laws prevent medical tasks from being performed by providers living in other states or countries. Foreign physicians also lack the authority to order certain tests, initiate therapies and prescribe drugs that American pharmacies can legally dispense.

States license and regulate physicians with the ostensible goal of maintaining the quality of medical care. However, state medical boards are dominated by physicians and, like the boards governing other regulated professions, they tend to benefit the practitioners. Besides stringent licensing requirements, these organizations suppress competition among physicians by declaring certain practices to be unethical. Medical societies have long opposed innovations that pose a threat to their autonomy or income. And threats to hospital revenue or the ability of hospital systems to cross-subsidize uncompensated care generate considerable opposition.

Some restrictions on the practice of medicine have been removed in recent years, but many still exist. For example:

— It is illegal for a physician to consult with a patient online without an initial face-to-face meeting.

— It is illegal in most states for a physician outside the state who has examined a patient in person to continue treating the patient via the Internet after the patient returns home.

— It is illegal in most states for a physician outside the state to consult by phone with patients residing in the state if the physician is not licensed to practice medicine there.

These laws make it difficult for American patients to seek care from doctors abroad via telephone and the Internet.

Restrictions on Collaboration among Health Care Providers

A physician practice in the United States could easily provide doctor visits in a traditional office, coupled with chronic disease management services from a foreign doctor and tests done at a convenient retail clinic when needed. Yet this scenario might run afoul of the so-called Stark Laws - 42 U.S.C. § 1395nn (b) (Medicare), § 1396 n(b) (Medicaid) (1982). The federal Stark laws make it illegal for a physician to refer a patient for treatment to a clinic in which the doctor has a financial interest. It is also illegal for a physician to reward providers who refer patients to him, or to a hospital in which he has a financial interest. Unfortunately, laws meant to prevent self-dealing and kickbacks also inhibit beneficial collaboration between doctors and hospitals. For instance, the Stark laws could prevent a physician practice from referring a patient with a chronic condition to an affiliated disease management program (employing a foreign doctor) or prevent the practice from referring a patient needing minor treatment to an affiliated walk-in clinic. By limiting compensation arrangements for referrals and collaboration, the Stark laws tend to result in rigid physician group practices that are not particularly convenient or economical for patients.

Lack of Follow-Up Care

Some procedures require follow-up care to monitor the healing process or remove stitches, for example, case of Betty Meisel cosmetic surgery gone wrong Bumrungrad International Hospital Bangkok. In some cases, patients who have travelled abroad for medical procedures have problems finding a local physician willing to provide postoperative follow-up care. "Aftercare is one of the most important issues and problems in medical tourism," said Jonathan Edelheit, president of the Medical Tourism Association. This is especially worrisome if the patient has complications. Liability for another provider's work is a perceived risk to doctors providing after care one reason some American physicians are loath to provide follow-up care to patients treated abroad.

Another reason for physicians' reluctance to provide follow-up care is that patients treated abroad often lack insurance. Over the years, many doctors have assumed that health insurance is the only way for patients to finance medical care. Physicians may prefer not to treat uninsured patients (unless payment is made in advance) for fear they will not get paid. Although lack of follow-up care is definitely a concern, many patients who have surgery abroad arranged in advance, perhaps report their regular doctor continued to treat them throughout recovery. Patients with a regular physician will likely fare better than those who are only seeking physician care for a short-term (postoperative) need.

Legal Obstacles

Employers and insurers could lower health costs by sending employees abroad for treatment. However, there are important legal considerations. Plan sponsors must meet Employee Retirement Income Security Act (ERISA) fiduciary obligations in designing and managing employee benefit plans. According to some legal scholars, an employer that sponsors a health plan offering workers a financial incentive to travel abroad for treatment could have greater liability risks. The concern is that financial incentives might induce enrollees to accept substandard care when they otherwise would select the local hospital of their choice although many health plans do just that by offering financial incentives for patients to choose hospitals in their networks. If health plans cannot offer enrollees financial incentives, patients are unlikely to consider medical travel.

Federal and State Government Plan Obstacles

Nearly half of all health care expenditures in the United States are paid for by the government; this includes Medicare, Medicaid and health coverage for state and federal workers. It is hard to imagine significant cost savings occurring without involving the public sector.

Medicaid consists of 50 different state programs. State Medicaid programs near the border with Mexico could easily outsource some procedures abroad. Yet despite the potential savings for state taxpayers, none have considered taking this step. Medicare benefits are limited to the United States. This is a hardship on foreign-born workers who accrue benefits in the United States but want to return to their homelands to retire. This also forces the estimated 40,000 to 80,000 American retirees living in Mexico to pay out of pocket or return to the United States to receive care. Furthermore, Medicare requires significant patient cost-sharing, generally twenty percent above the deductible. Medicare could reduce costs and allow seniors to share in the savings by waiving the cost sharing requirements.

Policy Solutions

The first step is for state and federal policymakers to understand that global competition in health care will benefit American consumers by reducing costs and improving quality through competition. Just as global competition improved the quality of automobiles; it will also improve the quality of medical care. Local politicians and community activists often fight to protect community hospitals from closure in the belief that communities cannot do without them. However, lawmakers must take advantage of cost-saving techniques in health care.

Modernize State Licensing Laws

Medical licensing laws must conform to the information age, where distance is irrelevant. Reforms should include recognizing standards of other countries as an alternative to local licenses. For instance, many Indian and Thai physicians are board-certified or licensed in the United Sates, Australia, Britain or Canada. Foreign physicians who meet standard criteria should be considered licensed if their skills have been evaluated and approved for inclusion in a network. It does not make sense in the information age for each state to approve and police physicians living thousands of miles away. The same holds true for physicians practicing in the United States. Laws that prevent physicians in one state from consulting with patients in other states by telephone or e-mail should also be eased.

Relax Laws Restricting Collaboration

The federal Stark laws prohibiting self-referral should be modified to allow beneficial arrangements where care is coordinated and provided in a more efficient manner. Without revised legislation, it would be difficult to integrate the services of physicians living abroad into the practices of local providers. Integrated medical services would also allow domestic providers to compete by creating more efficient operations. For example, a traditional physician practice could offer disease management for chronic conditions at a lower cost through an associated Indian physician. And an American radiologist might have an Indian radiologist read X-rays at costs lower than competitors.

Encourage Follow-Up Care

While physicians prefer an ongoing relationship with a patient, outsourcing patients to providers abroad is not much different than referring them to a specialist down the street. If "safe harbour" contracts were created for physicians providing follow-up care, more doctors would be willing to treat cash-paying patients. Moreover, if the number of medical tourists rises significantly, entrepreneurial physicians and clinics will sense an opportunity to provide follow-up care. To facilitate providing follow-up care for patients who return from treatment abroad, a committee of the American Medical Association has recommended creating a current procedural terminology (CPT) reimbursement code for patients who need postoperative follow-up care.

Facilitate Liability by Contract

Some American patients may be concerned about the potential difficulty of holding providers accountable in foreign legal systems and of receiving compensation for complications that will undoubtedly arise from medical treatment abroad. Federal law needs to recognize patient contracts that provide for binding arbitration or that limit liability. For instance, patients could purchase additional insurance from their health insurer in an amount they believe will protect them in the event of predefined problems that might occur from foreign treatment. A policy could clearly identify financial remedies for specific problems similar to an accidental death and dismemberment policy, for example, life insurance policies.

Allow Financial Incentives

Lately, some insurers have begun creating low-cost health plans that rely on foreign-based providers to treat serious ailments.

Unfortunately, lawyers could interpret ERISA and Health Insurance Portability and Accountability Act of 1996. ("HIPAA" - 42 U.S.C. § 1320) regulations in ways that discourage employers (and health plans) from providing patients with financial incentives to travel abroad for lower-cost care. Insurers and self-insured employers should have the right to experiment with a range of health benefits that inject global competition into health care. In addition, insurers, health plans and self-insured employers that have facilitated the overseas treatment of willing patients should be protected from liability.

Medical tourism is likely to increase over the next decade as more patients are able to access the Internet and acquire information relevant to care offered overseas at an affordable price. While some patients will benefit immensely from treatment as a medical tourist, many legal and ethical issues will also arise. Health care professionals need to familiarize themselves with the benefits of medical tourism while also acknowledging its inherent dangers. Potential medical tourists will benefit from the services of a knowledgeable health professional in their home country who can discuss the many issues that relate to this medical tourism. It is expected that medical tourism will provide a new role for health care professional as this health care trend expands around the world.

References

Borman, E. (2004). Health tourism: Where health care ethics and the state collide. *British Medical Journal*, 328, 60–61.

Brady, C.J. (2007), "Ofshore Gambling: Medical Outsourcing Versus ERISA's Fiduciary Duty Requirement", Washington & Lee Law Rev. 64 (3), 1073-1114.

Chaynee, W. (2003). *Health tourism to drive earnings*. Kuala Lumpur: Malaysian Institute of Economic Research.

Case of Bety Meisel. (2008): "Cosmetic Surgery Gone Wrong", *The Washington Post*, July 2008 http://www.washingtonpost.com/

De Arelano, A.B.R. (2007). "Patient Without Borders: The Emergence of Medical Tourism ", *International Journal of Health Services*. 37 (1), 193-198.

Gray, H.H. and S.C. Poland. (2008), "Medical Tourism : Crossing Boarders to access healthcare", *Kennedy Institute of Ethics Journal*. 18(2), 193-201.

Howze, K.S. Spring (2007), Medical Tourism: Symptom or Cure?, *Ga Law Rev.* 41 (3), 1014-1050.

Jones, C.A. and L.G. Keith. (2006), "Medical Tourism and Reproductive Outsourcing: the Drawing of a New Paradigm for Healthcare", *Int J Fertil.* 51 (6), 251- 255.

Mattoo, A. and R. Rathindran. (2006), " How Health Insurance Inhibits Trade In Health Care", *Health affairs* (Millwood). 25:358-368

Reed, CM,. (2008). "Medical Tourism," *Medical Clinics of North America*, Vol 92, No 6, pp. 1433 .

Smerd Jeremy. (2008). Large Companies hopping aboard medical tourism, *Workforce Management* June 23, Vol 87. Issue 11, p. 8 10.

Woodman, Josef. (2008). *Patients Beyond Borders: Affordable World Class Medical Travel*, Healthy Travel Media, Chapel Hill, North Carolina.

Bibliography

Arellano ABR. (2007). Patients Without Borders: The Emergence of Medical Tourism. *International Journal of Health Services* 37(1):193–198.

Arunanondchai, Jutamas and Carson Fink, (2006)."Trade in Health Services in the ASEAN region," *Health Promotion International,* Vol. 21 pp. 59-66.

Avigail M. Olarte, (2006). "Health and the Philippines: And now hospitals as tourist spots", *Philippines Center for Investigative Journalism*, 12 September.

Bartha M. Knoppers & Sonia LeBris, (1991). Recent Advances in Medically Assisted Conception: Legal, Ethical, and Social Issues, 17 *Am. J.l.&Med.* 329, 333.

Bennett, M.; King, B. and Milner, L. (2004). "The health resort sector in Australia: A positioning study", *Journal of Vacation Marketing.* vol.10, no.2, pp.122-137.

Bookman and Bookman. (2007). *Medical Tourism in Developing Countries* New York: Palgrave Macmillan.

Bookman MZ, Bookman KR. (2007). *Medical Tourism in Developing Countries*. New York: Palgrave Macmillan.

Bookman, Milica Z. and Karla R. Bookman, (2007).*Medical Tourism in Developing Countries*, Palgrave Macmillan, NY.

Borman, E. (2004). Health tourism: Where health care ethics and the state collide. *British Medical Journal*, 328, 60–61.

Brady, C.J. (2007), "Ofshore Gambling: Medical Outsourcing Versus ERISA's Fiduciary Duty Requirement", Washington & Lee Law Rev. 64 (3), 1073-1114.

Canales, MT, BL Kasiske, ME Rosenberg, (2007)."Transplant Tourism: Outomes of United States Residents Who Undergo Transplantation Overseas," *Transplantation,* Vol 82, No. 12, 1858-1862.

Case of Bety Meisel. (2008): "Cosmetic Surgery Gone Wrong", *The Washington Post,* July 2008 http://www.washingtonpost.com/

CBS (2004). "Medical tourism: Need surgery, will travel", *CBS News Indepth*: healthcare, June 18,2004.

Cetron , M. .De Micco, F.J. and Davies, O. (2005) *Hospitality 2010: The Future of Hospitality and Travel,* Forecasting International , USA

Chaynee, W. (2003). *Health tourism to drive earnings*. Kuala Lumpur: Malaysian Institute of Economic Research.

Connell J. (2006). Medical tourism: Sea, sun, sand and ... surgery. *Tourism Management* 27:1093–1100.

Cortez, Nathan, (2008)."Patients Without Borders: The Emerging Global Market for Patients and the Evolution of Modern Health Care," *Indiana Law Journal*, Volume 83: pp. 71-132.

Crell, G.A.C., (1994). "Ecotourism and Health Tourism in the Caribbean," *Bulletin of Eastern Caribbean Affairs*, pp. 39-45 .

Dastur, A. (2005). Umblical cord blood banking, *Journal of Obstetrics and gynecology of India,* Vol. 55, no. 6.

David Diaz Benavides, (2002). "Trade policies and export of health services: a development perspective" in Vieira Cesar ed., *Trade in Health Services: Global, Regional and Country Perspectives* . Washington D.C., PAHO.

De Arelano, A.B.R. (2007). "Patient Without Borders: The Emergence of Medical Tourism ", *International Journal of Health Services*. 37 (1), 193-198.

Deloitte. (2008). *Medical Tourism. Consumers in Search of Value*. Washington DC: Deloitte Centre for Health Solutions.

Diana M. Ernst, (Sept. 2006). Medical Tourism: Why Americans Take Medical Vacations Abroad, 4 *Pac. Res. Inst.* 1.

Douglas, N., Douglas, N. and Derrett, R. (2001). *Special Interest Tourism*, Wiley, Australia

Edwin Borman, (2004). Health Tourism: Where Healthcare, Ethics, and the State Collide, 328 *Brit. Med. J.* 60, 60.

ESCAP. (2009). *Medical Travel in Asia and the Pacific. Challenges and Opportunities*. Bangkok: United Nations Economic and Social Commission for Asia and the Pacific.

Fisher, G.; Hughes, R.; Griffin, R. and Pustay, M. (2006). *International Business* Prentice Hall, Frenchs Forest.

Frechtling, D.C. (1997). "Current research on health and tourism issues and future directions," in *Tourism and Health: Risks, Research, and Responses*, Clift, S. and Grabowski, P. eds., Pinter, London.

Ganapati Mudur, (2004). Hospitals in India Woo Foreign Patients, 328 *Brit. Med. J.* 1338, 1338.

Garcia-Altes, M. (2005). "The development of health tourism services", *Annals of Tourism Research*, vol.32, no.1,pp.222-266.

Government, Private Sector Chart Medical Tourism Direction, Business World. Manila. (2007).

Gray, H.H. and S.C. Poland. (2008), "Medical Tourism : Crossing Boarders to access healthcare", *Kennedy Institute of Ethics Journal*. 18(2), 193-201.

Gupta Sen Amit, (2004). "Medical Tourism and Public Health", *People's Democracy*, 9 May, Vol. XXVIII No. 19

Henderson, J.C. (2004). "Healthcare tourism in Southeast Asia", *Tourism Review International*, vol.7, pp.111-121.

Herrick DM. 2007. Medical Tourism: Global Competition in Health Care. *NCPA Policy Report No. 304*, November 2007.

Hope-Price, G. (1994). *Health Tourism*, Prepared for the World Bank, Dover Convention Centre, Barbados, December 15.

Howze, K.S. Spring (2007), Medical Tourism: Symptom or Cure?, *Ga Law Rev*. 41 (3), 1014-1050.

Hutchinson, B. (2005). *Medical Tourism growing worldwide*, UDaily./ University of Delawre.

Johanna Paola D. Poblete, (2007). Special Feature: Medical Tourism, *Bus. World*, Philippines.

Jones, C.A. and L.G. Keith. (2006), "Medical Tourism and Reproductive Outsourcing: the Drawing of a New Paradigm for Healthcare", *Int J Fertil*. 51 (6), 251-255.

Lautier, Marc, (2008)."Export of Health Services from Developing Countries: The Case of Tunisia," Social Science and Medicine, 67, pp.101-110.

Linda F. Powers, (2006). Leveraging Medical Tourism, *The Scientist*, March

Malathy Iyer. (2004). "India Out to Heal the World," Times of India, October 26.

Marcelo, R. (2003). India Fosters Growing 'Medical Tourism' Sector, *The Financial Times*, July.

Mattoo, A. and R. Rathindran. (2006), " How Health Insurance Inhibits Trade In Health Care", *Health affairs* (Millwood). 25:358-368

Nicolas P. Terry, (2007), Under-Regulated Healthcare Phenomena in a Flat World: Medical Tourism and Outsourcing, 29 *W. New Eng. L. Rev*. 421

Philip Stevens, (2005)*Free trade for better health*. London, International Policy Network.

Prasad, R. (2004) Cord Blood:Biolcgical Insurance, SciTech- Online Edition of The Hindu .

Prosenjit Datta and Gina S. Krishnan, (2003). "The Health Travellers", *BusinessWorld*, 22 December, accessed from <http://www.business worldindia.com/issue/pharma.asp>.

Rajghatta, C. (2007). Medical Tourism: Idiomatical American Sicko can reach out to India, by Knight Ridder, *Tribune Business News*. Washington.

Ray Marcelo, (2003). "India Fosters Growing 'Medical Tourism' Sector", *The Financial Times*, 2 July, accessed from <http://yaleglobal.yale.edu/display.article?id=2016>

Reed, CM,. (2008). "Medical Tourism," *Medical Clinics of North America*, Vol 92, No 6, pp. 1433 .

Shepard, D.S. and Vargas, V. (1995). *Health Tourism in Barbados: A Preliminary Assessment*, mimeograph, February 16.

Smerd Jeremy. (2008). Large Companies hopping aboard medical tourism, *Workforce Management* June 23, Vol 87. Issue 11, p. 8 10.

Smith K. (2008). Medical Tourism: For Richer or Poorer. *Paper presented at Ownership & Appropriation, a joint conference of the ASA, the ASAANZ and the AAS*, 8th - 12th December 2008, University of Auckland, New Zealand.

Smith, C. and Jenner, P. (1998). "The Senior's Travel Market," in Travel and Tourism Intelligence, *The Economist Intelligence Unit*.

Suwit Wibulpolprasert et al, (2004). "International service trade and its implications for human resources for health: a case study of Thailand", *Human Resources for Health*, Vol. 2, No. 10

UNCTAD-WHO Joint Publication, (1998). *International Trade in Health Services: A Development Perspective,* Geneva, Switzerland.

Warner, D.C., (1998). "The Globalization of Medical Care," in UNCTAD-WHO Joint Publication, *International Trade in Health Services: A Development Perspective*, Geneva, Switzerland.

Watt, P. and Davis,.G. (2003) *Scenario : An Explorers' Guide* , Shell International Ltd, London

Wee Sui Lee, (2007). "Medical tourism boosts Asian hospital shares", *The Bangkok Post*, 23 June.

WHO (2000). *The World Health Report 2000 – Health Systems: Improving Performance*. Geneva: WHO.

Woodman, J. (2007). *Patients Beyond Borders-Everybody's Guide to Affordable World Class Medical Tourism;* Catanoba Publishing, USA.

World Bank, (1993). *World Development Report: Investing in Health*, Washington, D.C. 1993.

Index